WOMEN

★ TO THE ★

FRONT

Heather Sheard is a former Victorian secondary school teacher and assistant principal. After retiring, she researched the history of Victoria's Maternal & Child Health Centres for a Master's degree at the University of Melbourne, published as *All the Little Children: The Story of Victoria's Baby Health Centres* in 2007 and reprinted in 2017. Her PhD, also undertaken at the University of Melbourne was a biography of Dr Vera Scantlebury Brown, published in 2016 as *A Heart Undivided: The Life of Dr Vera Scantlebury Brown, 1889–1946*. During her PhD research she was captivated by the stories of a number of largely unheralded Australian women doctors who served during the Great War, and determined to write about their experiences and contributions.

Heather has written articles for *The Conversation*, *Spirit of Progress*, *City of Kingston* and *Chiron* and chapters in *Founders, Firsts and Feminists: Women Leaders in Twentieth Century Australia*, 2011; *Strength of Mind: 125 Years of Women in Medicine*, ed. 2014 and 'Women Doctors: Proving their Worth' in *Compassion and Courage: Doctors and Dentists at War*, 2015.

Heather lives in Elwood, Victoria and has a 'petite' holiday cottage near the wineries of Burgundy, France.

Ruth Lee has taught Australian history and academic writing at Deakin University, Geelong for 25 years; her major research interest has been documenting women's history. Researching the life of Dr Mary De Garis, she was awarded her PhD at Deakin University in 2011 and went on to write the biography *Woman War Doctor: The Life of Mary De Garis*, which was commended by the Royal Historical Society of Victoria's Community History awards, Centenary of World War One category, 2015.

She has contributed articles to the University of Melbourne's Medical History Museum exhibition catalogues: *Strength of Mind: 125 Years of Women in Medicine*, ed. 2014 and 'Women Doctors: Proving their Worth' in *Compassion and Courage: Doctors and Dentists at War*, 2015; and biographical entries to *The Encyclopedia of Women and Leadership in Twentieth-Century Australia* (online) (2014).

Ruth lives on the Bellarine Peninsula in Victoria.

WOMEN

★ TO THE ★

FRONT

THE EXTRAORDINARY **AUSTRALIAN** **WOMEN DOCTORS** of THE **GREAT WAR**

HEATHER SHEARD
AND RUTH LEE

EBURY
PRESS

An Ebury Press book

Published by Penguin Random House Australia Pty Ltd
Level 3, 100 Pacific Highway, North Sydney NSW 2060
penguin.com.au

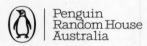

Penguin
Random House
Australia

First published by Ebury Press in 2019
Copyright © Heather Sheard and Ruth Lee 2019

A catalogue record for this
book is available from the
National Library of Australia

ISBN 978 0 14379 470 7

Cover images courtesy of University of Melbourne Archives (Dr Vera
Scantlebury Brown), Australian War Memorial (Dr Phoebe Chapple),
William Girling (Dr Kate Ardill) and Shutterstock
Cover design by Louisa Maggio © Penguin Random House Australia Pty Ltd
Typeset in 11/16.5 pt Janson Text by Post Pre-press, Brisbane
Printed in Australia by Griffin Press, an accredited ISO AS/NZS 14001:2004
Environmental Management System printer

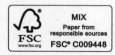

Contents

Medical and military abbreviations

AAMC	Australian Army Medical Corps
AIF	Australian Imperial Force
BFH	British Field Hospital for Belgium; sometimes called Belgian Field Hospital
CBE	Commander of the British Empire
CO/OC	Commanding Officer/Officer Commanding
EEF	Egypt Expeditionary Force
FANY	First Aid Nursing Yeomanry
FRCS	Fellow of the Royal College of Surgeons
HMATS	His Majesty's Australian Troop Ship
HMHS	His Majesty's Hospital Ship
HMTS	His Majesty's Troop Ship
LMSSA	Licentiate in Medicine and Surgery of the Society of Apothecaries
LRCP	Licentiate in the Royal College of Physicians and Surgeons
LSMW	London School of Medicine for Women
MB, BS/MB, ChB/ MB, ChM	Bachelor of Medicine, Bachelor of Surgery
MD	Doctor of Medicine, postgraduate qualification equivalent of Doctor of Philosophy
MO/CMO/SMO	Medical Officer/Chief Medical Officer/Senior Medical Officer
NUWSS	National Union of Women's Suffrage Societies
NZAMC	New Zealand Army Medical Corps
OBE	Order of the British Empire
QMAAC	Queen Mary's Army Auxiliary Corps
RAMC	Royal Army Medical Corps
RMS	Royal Mail Ship
SS	Steam Ship or Steam Screw
SWH	Scottish Women's Hospitals
VAD	Voluntary Aid Detachment
WAAC	Women's Army Auxiliary Corps
WARC	Wounded Allies' Relief Committee
WHC	Women's Hospital Corps
WO	British War Office
WRAF	Women's Royal Airforce

Australian women doctors known to have served in World War I

NAME (MARRIED NAME)	YOB–YOD	AGE IN 1914	EDUCATION (UNIVERSITY WHERE QUALIFIED, DEGREE, YEAR)	YEARS AND LOCATION OF SERVICE	MEDALS AWARDED
Dr Katie Ardill (Brice) OBE (1941)	1886–1955	28	University of Sydney, MB, ChM 1913	September 1915–February 1916, Anglo–Belgian Hospital, Calais, France; February 1916–January 1917, County of Middlesex War Hospital, Napsbury, Middlesex, England; February 1917–May 1918, Dover Military Hospital, England; May 1918–July 1919, Citadel Hospital, Cairo, Egypt; returned October 1919	British Red Cross Medal
Dr Ethel Baker	1885–1965	29	University of Brussels, MB, BS 1913	September–October 1914, Belgian Field Hospital, Belgium	British War Medal; Victory Medal, British Star
Dr Eveline Benjamin (Cohen)	1879–1922	35	Edinburgh College of Medicine for Women, MB 1909; University of Dublin, FRCS 1910	September 1916–September 1917, RAMC, Malta; November 1918–December 1918, Cambridge Military Hospital, Aldershot, England	

NAME (MARRIED NAME)	YOB–YOD	AGE IN 1914	EDUCATION (UNIVERSITY WHERE QUALIFIED, DEGREE, YEAR)	YEARS AND LOCATION OF SERVICE	MEDALS AWARDED
Dr Agnes Bennett OBE (1948)	1872–1960	42	University of Sydney, BSc, 1894; Edinburgh College of Medicine for Women, MB, ChM 1899, MD 1911	May 1915–May 1916, NZAMC, Egypt; August 1916–October 1917, SWH, Macedonia; 1918 Troopship, Royal Infirmary, Glasgow, Scotland; Welsh Military Hospital, Southampton, England	Order of St Sava, 3rd Class; Royal Red Cross of Serbia; British and French Red Cross Medals; Victory Medal
Dr Eleanor Bourne	1878–1957	36	University of Sydney, MB, ChM 1903 (10th female graduate)	May 1916–late 1917, Endell St Military Hospital, London, England; 1917–1918, WAAC (later QMAAC) Northern Area Medical Controller, York, England	
Dr Emma Buckley (Turkington)	1879–1959	35	University of Sydney, MB, ChM 1911	1915–1916, Lister Institute, London, England; 1916–1917, King George Military Hospital, London, England; briefly 1916–1917, Endell St Military Hospital, London, England; 1917–1918, King George Military Hospital	
Dr Hilda Bull (Esson, later Dale)	1886–1953	28	University of Melbourne, MB, ChB 1913	1917–1919, WAAC (later QMAAC), London, England	
Dr Rachel Champion (Shaw)	1890–1965	24	University of Melbourne, MB, ChB 1914	1916–1917, Endell St Military Hospital, London, England; briefly 1918, WAAC, London, England	

NAME (MARRIED NAME)	YOB–YOD	AGE IN 1914	EDUCATION (UNIVERSITY WHERE QUALIFIED, DEGREE, YEAR)	YEARS AND LOCATION OF SERVICE	MEDALS AWARDED
Dr Phoebe Chapple	1879–1967	35	University of Adelaide, BSc 1898; MB, BS 1904	1917, RAMC, Cambridge Military Hospital, Aldershot, England; November 1917–August 1918, WAAC (later QMAAC), Abbeville, Rouen, Le Havre, France	Military Cross (awarded Military Medal instead); British War Medal; Victory Medal
Dr Lilian Cooper	1861–1947	53	London School of Medicine for Women, MB, ChM, LRCP 1890; University of Durham, MD 1912	September 1916–August 1917, SWH, Macedonia	Order of St Sava, 4th Class; Russian decoration; French Red Cross Medal
Dr Grace Cordingley (Bridge)	1876–1969	38	University of Sydney, BArts 1898, MA 1903; London School of Medicine for Women, LMSSA 1913	1915–1918, Royal Free Hospital – Military Block, London, England	
Dr Elsie Dalyell OBE (1919)	1881–1948	33	University of Sydney, MB, ChM 1910	February–July 1915, Serbian Relief Fund field hospital (Lady Wimborne Unit), Serbia; July 1915–April 1916, Addington Park Military Hospital, Croydon, England; May–October 1916, SWH, Abbaye de Royaumont, France; October 1916–June 1917, RAMC, Malta; June 1917–1919, 63rd Hospital, Salonica, Greece; 1919, 82nd Hospital, Constantinople, Turkey	English and French Red Cross Medals; Mentioned in Dispatches twice; OBE for war work

NAME (MARRIED NAME)	YOB–YOD	AGE IN 1914	EDUCATION (UNIVERSITY WHERE QUALIFIED, DEGREE, YEAR)	YEARS AND LOCATION OF SERVICE	MEDALS AWARDED
Dr Mary De Garis	1881–1963	33	University of Melbourne, MB, BS 1905, MD 1907	October–December 1916, Manor Hospital, London, England; February 1917–September 1918, SWH, Macedonia	Order of St Sava, 3rd Class; French Red Cross Medal; British War Medal; Victory Medal
Dr Irene Eaton	1882–1920	32	London School of Medicine for Women, MB, ChM 1909	1916, Norfolk War Hospital; November 1916–October 1917, RAMC, Malta; October 1917–June 1919, WAAC (later QMAAC) Eastern Area Medical Controller, England	
Dr Letitia Fairfield CBE (1919)	1885–1978	29	Edinburgh College of Medicine for Women, MB, ChB 1907, MD 1911	1917–1918, Chief Medical Officer, Southern Command, WAAC; 1918–1919, Inspector of Medical Services, Women's Royal Air Force, London, England	
Dr Laura Forster	1858–1917	56	University of Bern, MB,ChM 1894, MD 1894	September 1914–early 1915, Belgian Field Hospital, Belgium; 1915–1917, St Petersburg Russian Red Cross, Caucasus, Russia; Millicent Fawcett Unit, Galicia Died of typhoid in Zaleschiki, Galicia, 29 January 1917	British War Medal; Victory Medal; British Star 1914–15
Dr Laura Fowler (Hope)	1868–1952	46	University of Adelaide, MB, BS 1891 (1st female graduate)	October 1915–February 1916, SWH, Serbia	Serbian Samaritan Cross

NAME (MARRIED NAME)	YOB–YOD	AGE IN 1914	EDUCATION (UNIVERSITY WHERE QUALIFIED, DEGREE, YEAR)	YEARS AND LOCATION OF SERVICE	MEDALS AWARDED
Dr Lucy Gullett	1876–1949	38	University of Sydney, MB, ChM 1901 (7th female graduate)	December 1915–May 1916, Red Cross, Egypt; June–December 1916, Hôpital d'Ulster, Lyon, France	French Red Cross Medal
Dr Lillias Hamilton	1858–1925	57	Edinburgh College of Medicine for Women and London School of Medicine for Women, MB, ChM, LRCP 1890; University of Brussels, MD c.1891	June–November 1915, WARC, Montenegro	British Red Cross Medal
Dr Elizabeth Hamilton-Browne MBE (1941)	1882–1985	30	University of Sydney, MB, ChM 1910	March 1916–March 1918, Endell St Military Hospital, London, England; 1918, No. 19 General Hospital, Egypt, Palestine	
Dr Marjory Little	1884–1974	30	University of Sydney, BSc 1911, MB, ChM 1915	June 1918–1919, RAMC, Rouen and Étaples, France	
Dr Mabel Murray-Prior	1882–1932	32	University of Sydney, 1903–1907, FRCS completed at University of Dublin, 1916; University of Edinburgh, MD 1917	1917, Royal Herbert Hospital, Woolwich, England; late 1918–1919, Edinburgh Hospital	

NAME (MARRIED NAME)	YOB–YOD	AGE IN 1914	EDUCATION (UNIVERSITY WHERE QUALIFIED, DEGREE, YEAR)	YEARS AND LOCATION OF SERVICE	MEDALS AWARDED
Dr Isabel Ormiston (Garvice) MBE (1928), OBE (1944)	1883–1958	31	University of Sydney, MB, ChM 1907	October–November 1914, early 1915, WARC, Belgium; May 1915–November 1915, WARC, Montenegro; briefly early 1916, British Convalescent Depot, Egypt; 1916–April 1918, WARC, Limoges, France	Mentioned in Dispatches; Montenegrin Red Cross; Order of Danilo; French Red Cross Medal
Dr Vera Scantlebury (Brown) OBE (1936)	1889–1946	25	University of Melbourne, MB, BS 1914, MD, 1924	May 1917–January 1919, Endell St Military Hospital, London, England	
Dr Helen Sexton	1862–1950	52	University of Melbourne, MB, BS 1892 (3rd female graduate)	July 1915–December 1915, Hôpital Australien, Auteuil, Paris; briefly Val de Grâce Hospital, Paris, France Major in French army	Gold Médaille de la Reconnaissance Française
Dr Isabella Younger (Ross) OBE (1938)	1887–1956	27	University of Melbourne and University of Glasgow, MB, ChB 1914	1916, Hospital for Belgian War Wounded, Kent, England	

Introduction

It is a curious mental astigmatism that allows a woman to work
with men on a hospital staff for years, and sends women nurses
to a base hospital, yet refuses women surgeons.[1]

Dr Helen Sexton, August 1915

World War I, known at the time as the Great War, was a humanitarian crisis of massive proportion. Lethal new technology that
killed and wounded people en masse joined with pandemic infections producing unprecedented loss of life and terrible affliction.
Hundreds of thousands fled, carrying disease with them while
also encountering new ones. Life in the war years was outside
everyone's previous experience and this unexpectedly allowed
women to circumvent some of the barriers faced pre-war; but not
without a struggle.

When the German army marched into Belgium in August
1914, Melbourne doctor Helen Sexton went straight to the British
War Office (WO) in London to offer her services to the Royal
Army Medical Corps (RAMC). At the time, 129 women were
registered as medical practitioners in Australia with around
1000 medical women in Britain, and many wanted to serve. For
military officialdom, however, the notion of women doctors
serving on the battlefield was outrageous. The answer throughout

the British Empire was an unequivocal 'No!'. Women doctors were not required for the war effort and advertisements were taken out to that effect in the newspapers.

But these were women accustomed to discouragement and to the denial of their professional capabilities. With routine determination and practised agility, at least twenty-six Australian women doctors ignored official military policy and served as surgeons, pathologists, anaesthetists and medical officers between 1914 and 1919. They served in Great Britain; on the Western Front in Belgium and France; on the Eastern Front including Serbia, Macedonia, Montenegro, Greece, Galicia and Russia; on the hospital island of Malta; and in Egypt and Palestine. *Women to the Front* is their story.

Women had pried open the doors of Australian medical schools twenty-five years before, with the first medical women graduating in 1891. Highly motivated and self-confident, they nevertheless needed a thick skin to succeed in qualifying and practising as doctors. Initially they had few role models and their experience at university and in postgraduate attempts to gain professional standing had deepened their feminist ideas and commitment to each other. However, in 1914 the acceptance of women into the medical profession remained tenuous. Their access to hospital residencies and the development of specialist medical skills, such as surgery, was extremely limited. In Melbourne this led to the creation of the Queen Victoria Hospital in 1896 for the provision of women doctors for women patients but also to provide valuable clinical experience for women doctors. Most practised within the sphere of women's and children's health and were referred to as 'lady doctors'. And 'lady doctors' did not go to war.

Yet the Great War's unrelenting need for medical services would clear the way for women doctors. Medicine was essential to war; it took centre stage in emergency treatment, in healing the wounded and sick, in health and hygiene for the armed services and in dealing with the dead. English doctor Flora Murray said that in August 1914, 'women doctors knew instinctively that the time had come when great and novel demands would be made upon them, and . . . an occasion for service was at their feet'.[2] Like their British counterparts, many Australian medical women saw the war as an extraordinary opportunity to validate their professional status by demonstrating their competence alongside their male peers in war.

Given the official discouragement, why did Australian women doctors want to go to war? Much of their motivation was the same as that of their male colleagues. They had been educated from childhood in a curriculum steeped in the centrality of the British Empire, its history and culture, and the need to contribute to the Empire's war effort was self-evident. They believed that it was their duty to use their medical training and experience to alleviate suffering, including on the battlefield. It is hardly surprising that many women wanted to share the patriotic burden of World War I with their brothers, fathers, uncles and fiancés serving overseas. The war provided a context, although a tragic one, of intensive clinical practice for medical personnel, and over its course ensured their exposure to the latest developments in medical research: infection control, blood typing and transfusion, the use of X-ray technology and new methods for saving damaged limbs. The chance to use and improve their medical skills was a professional opportunity that women doctors did not want to miss.

As the war kept on and on, it was also evident to women everywhere that the pre-war social mores proscribing their lives were weakening and that plentiful opportunities for personal agency could be seized. This was enormously appealing to women doctors who were accustomed to stretching the boundaries of social convention, especially when combined with the rare chance to work in surgery, pathology and orthopaedics outside the realm of women's and children's health. Women doctors were affected by the same contagious magnetism of travel and adventure that drew their male colleagues, as well as wanting to escape the humdrum, limiting predictability of their role as women doctors. Some may have feared being left standing on the sidelines rather than taking part in such a universal event. As May Sinclair, in Belgium in September 1914, wrote, 'If you miss it, you miss reality itself.'[3] Perhaps some women doctors dreamed of the chance to be heroic and to be recognised for it, however unrealistic this may have been.

The ages of the Australian women doctors who went to war varied from twenty-seven to fifty-six years and all but five were single women. They had been educated either at home or in private girls' schools and the support and encouragement of their families was fundamental. School and university fees were considerable and these women came from middle- and upper-class backgrounds.

Australian universities contributed fifteen of the women doctors but others had obtained their qualifications at the Edinburgh College of Medicine for Women, the London School of Medicine for Women (LSMW), and the universities of Bern, Brussels, Dublin and Glasgow. Six had completed their Doctor of Medicine (MD), the medical equivalent of a PhD, before undertaking their war service. Eleven of the women were inter-connected via Sydney Girls High School, the University of Sydney's Women's College and their studies at the University of Sydney. Five came from the University of Melbourne where the medical women were connected by their studies and their clinical experience at the Queen Victoria Hospital. The women had been a tiny minority in each of their medical student groups, relying principally on their female networks for affirmation. After graduation, the vicissitudes of life as a woman doctor, their professional isolation and sometimes the loneliness of their work situations encouraged their networks to continue and their letter-writing provided important news during the war years.

Germany invaded Belgium on 4 August 1914 and Britain immediately declared that it was at war with Germany. The conflagration that began was the first total war – one which engulfed not only opposing armies but civilian populations as well. The combatant armies had powerful new weaponry, which brought together a devastating combination of artillery using high explosives and machine guns. The effects on the human body were horrific, causing jagged wounds of all sizes often grossly contaminated. In the first months of the war, unprecedented mass casualties caused immense demand for medical staff and facilities. Civilian populations too were impacted by the rapid movement of the battle lines creating medical needs for which there were no plans. The static trench warfare on farmland that soon char-acterised the Western Front promoted dangerous infections such as gas gangrene in wounds, as well as typhoid and dysentery from prolonged close living. As the armies moved and civilians fled, infectious diseases thrived and added further medical complexity.

The scale of the casualties in the first months of the war resulted in a desperate scramble to put medical units into the field. This prompted the WO to create a Joint War Committee consisting of the British Red Cross and the Order of St John. The committee authorised voluntary medical units to go into the field. The volunteer units served on both the Eastern and Western Fronts throughout the war and Australian women doctors were welcomed. In the chaotic conditions that initially ensued, the volunteers established hospitals in Belgium and France in buildings hastily provided or commandeered and sent their newly fitted ambulances out to pick up wounded wherever they could find them. They pragmatically filled some of the yawning gaps in the under-resourced medical services during the first three or four months on the Western Front. Through the following four years of war they treated thousands of battle casualties and cared for civilian patients for whom governments made scarce provision.

On the Eastern Front, the need for medical resources was even more urgent and the means of transporting the wounded were often primitive. Austria–Hungary, an ally of Germany, crossed the Drina River invading Serbia on 12 August 1914. The Serbian army, still suffering the depletions of the First and Second Balkan Wars in 1912 and 1913, was undermanned and very poorly resourced in both armaments and medical services. By early 1915, a typhus epidemic, considered to be the worst in history, had broken out, claiming an estimated 150,000–200,000 lives in a population of 4.5 million. Voluntary medical units initially rushed to deal with the epidemic but found that wounded soldiers were lying beside typhus patients, both military and civilian.

Over the course of the war on the Eastern Front the battle lines moved with unpredictable and frightening fluidity. The women doctors of the voluntary units set up wherever an empty building was available and also worked in tented field hospitals under the same conditions as the combatants. When time allowed, they also treated civilians who were sometimes locals but also came from the tide of refugees that fled in front of advancing armies. The unprecedented scale of the war meant no real provision was made for sick or injured civilians affected everywhere by the conflict and the sudden dearth of medical services. Word always spread quickly of the presence of doctors and medicines, and mothers, in particular, brought their children to see the women doctors.

Other Australian women doctors joined medical organisations created under the banner of the women's suffrage movement in Britain, such as the Scottish Women's Hospitals (SWH), the Women's Hospital Corps (WHC) and the Millicent Fawcett Hospital Units. In 1914 British women still did not have the right to vote. Prominent women in the suffrage movement grasped the possibility of demonstrating their worthiness for citizenship by taking up war work. Pragmatically reshaping their campaign for the vote, the movement created military hospitals in London and France and sent mobile hospital field units, staffed almost entirely by women, right across the European battlefields. The hospitals and units were organised along military lines with uniforms designed for practicality and recognition and leaders referred to as Commanding Officer (CO) or Officer Commanding (OC) or Chief Medical Officer (CMO).

Another opportunity for women doctors came in mid-1916. The Battles of Verdun and the Somme were raging on the Western Front and the need for doctors was so great that women doctors were finally encouraged by the WO to work for the RAMC. However, this was to be a contractual arrangement and did not take the form of official enlistment. The women were given a rank only for the purpose of determining their salary. Their appointments were never gazetted and remained ex-officio until the end of the war. Officially, they did not hold a commission and were prohibited from wearing the badges and pips of their rank. This denied them the external symbols of authority and caused difficulty at times in carrying out their roles in a strictly hierarchical organisation. The Australian Army Medical Corps (AAMC) made no similar offer to Australian women doctors and, with the exception of a single letter, their service is unrecorded in the National Archives of Australia's World War I personnel records.

It must be acknowledged that we may never discover all of the Australian women doctors who went to war and we are also unable to chronicle the work of the women doctors who took over from their male colleagues on home fronts throughout the British Empire. The paucity of official records for the women featured in this book, and the lack of sources generally, has meant that while some women's experiences are relatively well documented, of others there are very few traces. We have only the letters, diaries and publications of a small number of the women and regret that this has led to some imbalances in the book's narrative. Any resulting errors of fact or interpretation are entirely our own. We look forward to receiving, through our publisher, information and corrections regarding the women we have written about and those we have yet to discover.

The small existing treasure trove of letters and diaries, however, does give us some idea of the women's emotions. Their writing, occasional sketches and photographs reveal excitement, wonder, satisfaction in duty done and the development of new skills, tempered by anxiety, frustration, exhaustion and the horror that was the Great War. The war confronted all doctors with dreadful wounds and highly infectious diseases, challenging their professional skills and their personal equanimity. A carapace of detachment was essential to survive the war's unrelenting provocation.

The journey was often fraught but the Australian women doctors who served overseas in the operating theatres and pathology labs of the Great War were able to find another version of themselves. This version is almost totally absent from official military records both in Australia and Great Britain and they have remained invisible for over a century. These women's stories reveal and honour their courage and commitment. Through narrating them here we provide some acknowledgement of the hundreds of lives they saved.

> On Friday, I operated and one man was so bad that I felt miserable . . . Thank heaven he is better this a.m.[4]
>
> Dr Vera Scantlebury, Endell Street Military Hospital, London,
> October 1918

Timeline and locations

The narrative of the women's war service follows roughly the timeline of World War I from 1914 to 1919. It is at best an inexact chronology of the war's evolution and is grounded in the reality of the women's day-to-day lives. Their war was tremendously uncertain, sometimes chaotic and without the structure and certainties with which we now view World War I.

Within each year the narrative is organised into five general locations:

The Western Front: This was a consolidation of the frontlines into a nearly unbroken line of trenches over a distance of more than 700 kilometres from the Belgian coastline in the north to the Swiss border in the south. Women doctors worked on the Western Front in voluntary hospital units and were permitted to work in RAMC hospitals in France from 1917.

The Eastern Front: This was more fluid and could shift rapidly as ground was taken, lost and retaken by both sides in the conflict. The front existed in discontinuous stretches for thousands of kilometres from Finland in the north to Macedonia in the south. In the northern part of the Eastern Front, Germany and Russia fought each other. In the southern part of the Eastern Front, the Austro–Hungarian Empire fought eastwards in Galicia against the Russians and southwards, invading Serbia, Macedonia and Montenegro. Women doctors worked in voluntary hospitals, sometimes in tents and often in very difficult conditions.

England/Scotland: Women doctors served in the hundreds of army hospitals and also voluntary hospitals established to treat the wounded and handle their convalescence.

Malta: The RAMC contracted women doctors to serve on the hospital island of Malta, strategically located in the Mediterranean, where they treated wounded and sick soldiers from the Dardanelles campaign and the Eastern Front.

Egypt: Cairo, Alexandria and Port Said were centres for medical treatment, initially for the casualties from the Dardanelles and later for the Middle Eastern campaigns, and women doctors worked in these cities throughout the war.

Part 1

1914

Chapter 1

'The War Office regrets'

The War Office regrets it cannot use the services of women doctors.[1]

Sydney Morning Herald, May 1915

I would gladly take war work if offered to me but so far my efforts have met no success . . . I think if the war continues, the need for doctors will be so great. That women will have a chance of being accepted and given military status for it.[2]

Dr Mary De Garis, Tibooburra, NSW, November 1915

Western Front: Antwerp, Belgium

September 1914, Autumn

'I hope to start for the front this week,' wrote Australian Dr Laura Forster to her sister in Sydney.[3] It was 31 August 1914 and Laura was writing from London where she had joined a voluntary hospital – the British Field Hospital for Belgium (BFH). Twenty-seven days earlier, six brigades of the Imperial German Army had crossed the eastern border of neutral Belgium, attacking the historic forts of the city of Liège, and Britain declared that it was at war with Germany. Two days later, on 6 August, the German army entered the forests of the Ardennes in north-eastern France.

This speedy double-pronged attack was the strategy of Germany's Schlieffen Plan with their armies moving westwards on two fronts to outflank the French. By the time Laura posted her letter to Australia, Liège's forts had been smashed and the German army had marched westwards, taking the Belgian cities of Namur on 25 August and Mons on 26 August.

In the Ardennes the French army was in retreat and headed for Verdun. The conflict was moving with unprecedented haste. In England the RAMC, as well as dozens of volunteer civilian units, rushed to organise hospital services in the field. By 5 September the BFH, including Laura, another Australian doctor Ethel Baker and English doctors Dorothea Maude and Alice Benham, were at sea. The unit was headed for Antwerp and the women were probably unaware that most of the Belgian army was now massed there and that the First German Army was moving swiftly northwards to conquer the city.

Laura was the daughter of Eliza Jane and William Forster, after whom the town of Forster in New South Wales is named. A tough and successful grazier, and a writer with a love of politics, William Forster was Premier of New South Wales for a short term and a politician of irascible independence for twenty-six years.[4] That independence was an evident trait in Laura, who had travelled to the University of Bern for her medical degree and in 1894 completed her MD on muscle spindle fibres. Known as a meticulous microscopist, Laura's first love, nevertheless, was surgery.

Ethel Baker was born in Queensland in 1885 but was barely six months old when her mother, Ethel Jemina, died. Her father, John Hamilton Baker, an architect and surveyor, remarried and, at the age of ten, Ethel was sent to live with her mother's family in London and the Isle of Wight. She gained her medical quali-fication at the University of Brussels, Belgium, and although she and her mother's family were pacifists she also saw merit in the concept of a 'just war' and wanted to do her duty. Ethel had a simple grey uniform made, wearing it with plain white shirts and an armband, no. 90899, issued by the Belgian Red Cross recog-nising her as a '*Docteur*'.

On 5 September, Laura and Ethel's volunteer unit boarded the *Marie Henriette*, a hastily commandeered Royal Mail paddle steamer, and a Red Cross yacht, the *Grace Darling*. A small British navy destroyer accompanied them, circling constantly like an anxious sheepdog. The group had gathered first at Victoria Station in London and then caused a sensation at the Kentish town of Folkestone, the English port closest to the war's frontline in Belgium.

The party was filmed as they stepped down from the train at the harbour station and marched out onto the quay.[5] The nine nurses were a striking sight in long violet cloaks with sky blue dresses, but it was the four 'lady farmers' who caused public consternation by daring to appear in what seemed to be men's trousers and long riding boots. They brought with them a large wagon and four-horse team but these were rapidly deemed unsuit-able and left behind on the wharf. The nurses, four male doctors, four female doctors, four drivers and four society ladies who had come along to assist made up the initial BFH. The crossing was rough, the paddle steamer sat low in the water and many passen-gers were seasick but the new unit's members were all hopeful that the chop would keep them safe from German submarines.[6]

The trip was not Laura's first into a war zone. The experience of war had made its first claim on Laura's sensibilities two years earlier in 1912. By that time the Ottoman Empire of the Turks was crumbling and on 8 October 1912 Montenegro declared war on their Ottoman rulers. Serbia, Bulgaria and Romania followed suit soon after, the four countries forming the Balkan League with the aim of pursuing independence from the Empire. The First and Second Balkan Wars were fought in 1912 and 1913 and, although Serbia conscripted at least eighty per cent of their 370 doctors, the demand for medical staff and supplies far outstripped their own capability.[7] The Serbian Red Cross asked for urgent assistance, and voluntary medical field units arrived from overseas, including England. Laura joined one of these units and was sent to Epirus, a rugged and mountainous region shared today between Albania and Greece.[8] Hundreds of battle casualties needed immediate medical treatment but, additionally, the eventual defeat of the Turks precipitated the movement of large numbers of ethnic Turkish refugees. Contagious diseases like typhoid spread easily and rapidly amongst the refugees and the armies.

Little is known about Laura's work in the Balkan Wars but the British Red Cross was one of the main suppliers of medical aid to the Balkan League and the organisation was unwilling to accept women as doctors in their units. Instead, Laura grasped the opportunity to go as a nurse and to experience the strange mixture of wounds and afflictions in both the military and the civilian populations in this region of contested ethnicity and religion.

Her first experience of war may have been the precedent for Laura's unhesitating approach two years later to the BFH in London in August 1914. A voluntary unit with the patronage of Queen Elisabeth of the Belgians and sanctioned by the British Red Cross, the field hospital was well equipped to set up a 150-bed facility close to the frontline. At fifty-six years of age and with her previous war experience, Laura was the matriarch of the women doctors. Alice Benham was forty-one, Dorothea Maude thirty-five and Ethel Baker had just turned twenty-nine and was about to face her first war wounds.

Laura and Ethel's unit landed at the Belgian port of Ostend, a holiday and casino resort on the northern Flanders coast. Before the war, Ostend was favoured by the European nobility and members of the English and Russian royal families strolled along its beachfront promenade. It was Belgium's largest coastal town and 120 kilometres from the fortified city of Antwerp – part of the war's frontline. After so much acclaim and excitement at Folkestone, their arrival in Belgium was subdued. Arriving before dawn in the rain, they wandered into Ostend's lofty glass-domed Central Station. It was completely deserted and, in the absence of a welcome, the group huddled together in the station's waiting room. All rail traffic had apparently been suspended and, anticipating a long delay, they removed the bright red plush cushions from a train carriage, laying them on the floor of the waiting room. Everyone slept on the velvet livery for the following two nights. On their third day a message from the Belgian queen told them to proceed on to Antwerp, and some of the BFH staff departed that evening by train.

The nurses anxiously watched them leave and worried that a wandering band of German light cavalry – Uhlans – would suddenly spring from the shadows and wipe them out. Next morning, Laura's party drove through the flat countryside of northern Flanders past the towns of Zeebrugge and Bruges and dozens of tiny Flemish villages. Villagers waved their caps and handkerchiefs and shouted *'Vive les Anglais!'* and the travellers shouted back *'Vive les Belges et à bas les Allemands!'*[9] Just before Ghent in the little town of Eecloo (Eeklo), Laura sighted her first evidence of war. A broad phalanx of soldiers marched grimly past wearing the long, dark blue greatcoats of the Belgian army. The travellers had seen few Belgian men. Only the women were working in the fields, tending cattle and driving market-carts and milk-carts with their polished brass cans.[10] The party's car trip ended in one of the great squares of Antwerp where people called out 'The English have come! The English have come!' and brought out wine and sandwiches.

Laura and Ethel's hospital was allocated one of the largest houses in Antwerp at 99 Boulevard Leopold, flanked by broad footpaths and the homes of the wealthy. A huge doorway opened into an outer hall, well suited to unloading stretchers, and a wide flight of white marble steps led to the great central hall of the building. Here they set up the largest wards with the operating theatre close by. The first floor and another above it were used as smaller wards, each containing from six to twelve beds. The Surgeon-in-Chief, Dr Henry Souttar, thought the light and airy house, most recently a school, was very suitable for a hospital of 150 beds but the nurses found the white marble staircases and working over four levels exhausting.

Hearing that the fighting was not far away, the staff unpacked dozens of crates and installed their equipment in three days. The German army was rapidly covering the distance between Mons and Antwerp and was now only 20 kilometres away at Malines (Mechelen). By around 13 September the hospital was ready and the BFH's motor ambulance headed out toward the fighting. In the first weeks of the conflict, arrangements for locating and picking up wounded soldiers were haphazard. Sometimes able-bodied soldiers carried the injured to the waiting ambulances; sometimes the drivers and doctors picked them up from the field.[11]

Laura, having already experienced war and triage nursing, was ready for these ventures into villages close to the heavy fighting. On their return, they described how Malines' magnificent St Rimbaut Cathedral had been badly damaged by German bombing, and its ancient stained-glass windows shattered. More disturbing were the shattered human beings they encountered. The civilian population received no warning of the bombings and on the ambulance's trip towards the fighting, the sights were unnerving even to the most experienced of the staff. World War I was the first war to target both military and civilian sites with large-scale artillery. There was very little forethought for the medical care of fleeing and wounded civilians, the victims of the bombardments. Both civilian and military casualties poured into central Antwerp.

The moment Laura and Ethel's hospital opened its doors, 170 wounded soldiers arrived, more than the hospital had beds for. All of the prepared wards, as well as the nurses' bedrooms and the larger landings, were immediately filled with beds and stretchers. Every one of the patients carried in on that first day was seriously wounded and the operating theatre's two tables were never empty, with the surgeons, including Laura and Ethel, working through the night. The nine nurses were scarcely able to keep abreast of the triage work and post-operative care. By three in the morning, many of the patients' wounds were dressed, and 'their poor mangled bodies resting'.[12]

Laura prized the practice of surgery and finally had the opportunity to use her skills. Women doctors in both Britain and Australia had only very limited access to surgical work and the tragic occurrence of war nevertheless provided intensive professional experience. Dr Souttar wrote that it was no use putting up a sign saying 'House Full' because, during their time in Antwerp, groups of wounded soldiers numbering from fifty to 150 were delivered without warning. Wounded soldiers had invariably lost blood, were suffering from shock and had certainly been lying anxiously for hours in pain, exposed to the weather and bombardment. They were firstly made warm and circulation restored with hot water bottles, blankets and brandy, and saved from pain and continued shock with morphia. Only then could the surgeons begin to deal with the wounds in the operating theatre.

In most cases the wounds of the soldiers who arrived on Laura and Ethel's operating tables were anything but clean-cut; with very few exceptions they were not surgically clean. Fractures of the leg were the most awkward for the surgeons to deal with and often involved a large infected wound and several inches of missing bone. These required a whole new range of surgical procedures, which Dr Souttar helped to develop over the war years. The work was heavy for everyone but particularly taxing for the nursing staff. Laura's previous wartime nursing provided her with a unique insight into the nurses' experience and they liked and respected her.[13] The beds were not regular hospital issue and were back-breaking, very low and with high iron sides. Many of the patients were solid men with septic wounds that had to be dressed several times a day, requiring the men to be lifted and turned. Laura was fifty-six years old in 1914 and of slight build but also indefatigably resolute in examining the wounds whilst leaning over the impractical beds. Ethel was twenty-seven years younger but was experiencing the trauma that came with a first exposure to war wounds and very shocked young men.

The sound of German artillery had grown steadily closer since the BFH's arrival in Antwerp, and on 29 September the Belgian army began preparations for the evacuation of their armaments, supplies and the wounded. The following day, the city's water supply failed. The waterworks at Waelhem, 6 kilometres south of the city, had been bombed extensively and hospital life became even more taxing. The local authority pumped water from the river for half an hour each day but it was brackish, salty and had to be boiled. When the water quickly became both undrinkable and unhealthy, many of the staff resorted to drinking beer. In Laura and Ethel's operating theatres the water was stored in large jugs but this frequently ran out when a rush of wounded arrived. Milk and butter supplies dwindled but, more importantly, so did Antwerp's population. The hospital's cooks disappeared as frightened Belgian families fled ahead of anticipated bombing and the stories of the atrocities of the invading German army.

With the arrival of a small force of British Royal Naval marines, the hospital was treating both Belgian and British wounded. Antwerp's ring of forts, the National Redoubt, was heavily bombed but Laura and Ethel's hospital continued its work to the background noise of artillery. The situation was rapidly becoming untenable and on 2 October the staff received their first notice to prepare for a likely evacuation. Laura would have been unaware that, eight days earlier, her half-brother Lionel had arrived at Le Mesnil, south of Antwerp, with the British army's Cheshire Regiment.

Western Front: Ostend, Belgium

September 1914, Autumn
Australian doctor Isabel Ormiston, from the New South Wales town of Albury, was working in the coastal city of Ostend and Belgian refugees had been fleeing to the city's port since the German invasion on 4 August 1914. Families were crammed into the dozens of tiny bathing boxes, crudely painted in blues, reds and

yellows, that were parked along Ostend's fashionable beachfront. Isabel could see the families from the casino-hotel, Le Kursaal, where she was in charge of a hospital newly created in the spacious ballroom. The spa hotel, with large gaming and ballrooms, sat along the beach promenade with an impressive facade of five towers, three domes and massive arched windows. It was not at all like the border town where Isabel grew up, which lay along the flat plains of the slow-moving Murray River that separated New South Wales from Victoria.

Along with the younger members of the large Ormiston family, Isabel was educated at Albury's Superior Public School, where she excelled academically. In her first year at the University of Sydney she studied Arts but, perhaps influenced by the professions of her four brothers, who were dentists and pharmacists, switched to a medical degree in 1902.

Isabel had joined the Wounded Allies' Relief Committee (WARC) at Sardinia House in London when war erupted. The British Red Cross had allocated the task of caring for Belgian wounded and refugees to the WARC, and in late September 1914 Isabel was appointed as the Medical Superintendent at Ostend's Le Kursaal.

Initially the converted casino-hotel was meant for sick and injured Belgian women and children. As Belgium's great forts fell to German shelling and the German army advanced, many Belgian people fled to Ostend in the hope of boarding a boat to England. They had been leaving Ostend for Dover and Folkestone by mail packets, fishing boats and any vessel they could board from the middle of August. In the first year of the war, around 160,000 Belgian refugees found shelter in Britain, where more than 2500 committees all around the country provided charitable relief to the arrivals.[14]

Isabel arrived in Ostend with an English nurse, Matron Monica Patton-Bethune from West Sussex. Monica was married to Major Douglas Patton-Bethune whose family from Burgess Hill on the edge of the South Downs had a long history of military careers. Married nurses could not enlist with the army medical corps and served instead with voluntary units like the WARC where they were gladly accepted. Isabel and Monica were initially in charge of fourteen staff and sixty beds. As the Belgian and French armies retreated, Le Kursaal swiftly became a military hospital and Isabel instantly had to turn her hand to military surgery.

By early October, Le Kursaal was inundated with wounded from the ever-changing frontline of the battles given the collective name of The Race to the Sea. The Allies were trying to prevent the German forces from reaching the coastal ports, including Ostend, because of their vital communication links with Britain. The wounded arrived at Isabel's hospital from the Battles of Artois, Arras, Messines and Armentières. The hospital's operating theatre was working in twenty-hour stretches as zeppelins attacked the Ostend railway station.[15] When they had any time to spare, Isabel and the nurses searched for a missing four-year-old boy. His mother had been brought to the hospital clasping a four-day-old baby and deranged after losing the little boy in the chaos – but no trace of him could be found.[16]

Laura Forster was still in Antwerp on Tuesday 5 October when hundreds of leaflets floated down from the sky warning that the German army would begin shelling Antwerp at midnight the following day. She had little time to read the airborne warnings. The hospital was working at capacity, evacuating any of the wounded who could possibly travel to make room for all the new wounded flooding in. The water situation was dire; the only positive for the nurses was that their workload was reduced because they were unable to maintain the daily washing of the white marble floors. Patients were washed only when absolutely necessary and water was limited to medical purposes, and for soup and coffee which barely disguised the terrible taste.

The boulevard in Antwerp where Laura and Ethel's hospital sat was a main road leading out through one of the great gates of the city. Throughout the next day, Wednesday 6 October, intense traffic noise infiltrated the wards. Cars drove by at top speed, heavy lorries lumbered past with a constant roar and the whole city appeared to be on the move. As Antwerp's city clock struck midnight:

We heard a boom far away, immediately followed by a new whistling scream increasing in volume and intensity till it became the roar of a train in a tunnel. It skimmed over our heads, literally raising our hair in its passage. This ended in a large, full explosion.[17]

Shells began to fall at two-minute intervals as the staff worked to empty the third floor of wounded. Fifty were placed on stretchers, along a network of underground passages and cellars. The work was done in darkness and when the wounded from all three floors were underground, strong sedatives were administered. The staff spent the rest of the night on the hard marble stairs. The noise was terrific, so they loudly sang 'Tipperary' and 'Dixie' and any other popular song they knew to drown out the explosions and mask their fear. The nurses appreciated Laura's sense of humour and that she could remain calm during the long uncomfortable night.[18]

Bombing continued through the night and as soon as first light dawned the staff began to evacuate the hospital. Eight motor omnibuses were borrowed from the British Marine Corps, their sides still pasted with the latest London music hall advertisements and displaying their original London destinations of Elephant & Castle and Hendon. Laura, Ethel and many of the staff and the wounded left the relative safety of their stone building to go out into the open street and sit waiting in the buses. Shells exploded in the hospital courtyard and crashed to the pavement nearby as nurses and doctors laboured to move their patients.[19] Those patients able to sit up were carried to the frighteningly open top level of the buses while stretcher cases were laid across the seats downstairs. The buses and five cars formed a long, slow procession as they moved erratically towards Ghent, 60 kilometres away. The trip took more than fourteen hours of terrible jolting as the buses lurched around bomb craters, rubble and refugees. The movement, combined with the pain from their wounds, caused many of the men to be violently sick. Dr Souttar wrote of that night:

> Of all the pitiful sights I have ever seen, that road was the most utterly pitiful. We moved on slowly through a dense throng . . . woman with three babies clinging to her skirts, a small boy wheeling his grandmother in a wheelbarrow, family after family, all moving away from the horror that lay behind to the misery that lay in front.[20]

The BFH convoy reached Ghent at dawn on Friday, but at 2 am on Saturday they were ordered to pack up and move again in order to stay ahead of the approaching German army. One soldier had died and two could not be moved from Ghent but everyone else, including Laura and Ethel, travelled the 60 kilometres in persistent and depressing drizzle, reaching Ostend at 4 am. Two

of the BFH's nurses begged a vacant bed at Isabel Ormiston's
Le Kursaal hospital for a quick nap. Several hundred wounded
had been delivered to the Kursaal's wards from Antwerp and
Ghent, adding to the numbers already there. The immense wards
were overflowing. Isabel had run short of anaesthetic and the
nurses heard 'lacerating' screams from the operating theatre.[21]

The evacuation process was chaotic as hundreds of
people – including Belgian and English wounded, medical
personnel and Belgian families – jostled to leave the port while
German planes intermittently bombed the harbour and nearby
sand dunes.[22] May Sinclair, an English writer who had gone to
Belgium with another volunteer unit, the Munro Ambulance
Corps, described the scene as one of

> most ghastly confusion . . . wounded lay wrapped in blankets
> on the terraces . . . ambulances jostled each other in the
> courtyard . . . Red Cross nurses with their luggage . . . a
> German bomb landed fifty feet away but did not explode.[23]

Laura and Ethel, with most of the other staff and patients of
the BFH's first mission, were loaded aboard ships returning to
England. Some of their wounded patients were lying below deck
in the saloon and cheered the BFH staff, relieved to see their
doctors and nurses had made it safely on board for the trip over
the water to Folkestone. Their boat was the second last to leave
Ostend before the Germany army took over the city.

Soon after Laura and Ethel had boarded the steamer for
England, Isabel Ormiston and Belgian doctor Emile Van de
Watte were on duty in the Le Kursaal hospital on 15 October,
as a 70,000-strong German army marched over the bridge that
spanned Ostend's harbour.[24] Isabel saw them arriving from a

balcony window and watched them set up a gun directly below, aimed at British warships in the harbour.[25] Immersed in surgery and the post-operative care of so many newly arrived wounded soldiers, Isabel, Monica and Emile refused to leave, although they were very unsure about how they would be viewed and treated by the Germans. Isabel and Monica became prisoners of the occupying army until late in October, when all British citizens were expelled from the Belgian coastal towns between Mariakerke, west of Ostend, and Knokke-Heist to the north. The German command believed that British spies in Ostend were providing information to the Royal Navy's warships that led to targeted firing on German positions. All British subjects were ordered to report to Ostend's Central Station and Isabel had no choice but to leave. Five train carriages were escorted under armed guard to the Dutch border and, by early November, Isabel was back in England.[26] She was 'mentioned in dispatches'[27] for gallant action in the face of the enemy.

Neither Laura Forster nor Isabel Ormiston remained in England for long. Belgium's Queen Elisabeth had formed a huge hospital in the small coastal village of La Panne (De Panne) behind the frontline at the river Yser, where the Belgian and French armies were holding on to a small remaining part of the country. Formerly the Grand Hotel de l'Ocean, the new L'Hôpital de l'Océan was intended for the severely wounded. The transformation of the hotel into a Red Cross hospital was the work of Dr Antoine DePage, a surgeon and head of the Belgian Red Cross.[28]

Back in England, Isabel Ormiston collected funds, motor vehicles and any medical equipment she could lay hands on and returned to Belgium to deliver them to La Panne.[29] At L'Hôpital, the patients bestowed the name *la petite docteuresse* on Isabel.[30]

Six kilometres away at Furnes (Veurne), the BFH returned in late October with new equipment and re-established its field hospital, setting up in a Catholic school. In their first four days, 350 wounded arrived from the Battle of Yser and conditions were grim. It is thought that Laura Forster was acting as anaesthetist and managing the unit's surgical equipment, which was in constant demand.[31]

By the end of October the Belgian army held only a small area along the coast between Nieuport (Nieuwpoort) and La Panne. On 28 October the Belgian defenders opened the floodgates at Nieuport. The city's complex canal system flooded the land and made the further advance of the German army impossible. The Belgian government and the royal family remained in La Panne for the duration of the war and this tiny part of Belgium remained at liberty.

London, England

August 1914, Summer
Melbourne doctor Helen Sexton had been travelling in England in August 1914 and had immediately put forward her surgical expertise to the RAMC, offering to pay all of her expenses and more. She brushed off their brisk refusal to enlist her. She tended to be rather brusque herself and had experienced refusal before. Helen determined to open her own hospital for '*les petits blessés*' in France, thus making her rejection by British military authorities irrelevant. She decided to return to Melbourne just as soon as she could get a homeward berth, and gather resources and people for a hospital. Within weeks, Helen was aboard the RMS *Moldavia*, a P&O mail and passenger ship sailing to Australia through

the Suez Canal. Her boat steamed past the SS *Kyarra* with the 1st Australian General Hospital on board, headed in the opposite direction to Helen and bound for Alexandria in Egypt. Aboard the *Kyarra* were many of Helen's recently enlisted male medical colleagues from Melbourne, some with far less surgical experience than her own.

She was back in Melbourne in early February 1915 and worked for almost four months raising money, gathering medical equipment and clothing (including 500 khaki handkerchiefs) and inspiring several women to help staff and fund her proposed hospital. By the end of May she was crossing back over the Indian Ocean on the RMS *Mooltan* with four of her friends and two nurses from Sydney's Royal Prince Alfred Hospital, all headed for Paris. The women were Susan Smith, her two daughters Alison and Lorna, Constance Blackwood, and nurses Florence Inglis and Dora Wilson. They were joined in France by Audrey and Eileen Chomley. Helen was a skilled surgeon and spoke good French and was readily offered a Parisian villa to set up her hospital by the French military. By July 1915 the hospital was open.

Part 2

1915

Chapter 2

'Beyond description'

The suffering of the sick and wounded and the appalling
waste of life here are beyond description.[1]

Dr Elsie Dalyell, Skopje, Serbia, March 1915

The war that was supposed to be over by Christmas swept on into
1915. The first Battle of Ypres in Belgium ended in late November
1914. Frost, early snow and rain slowed the fighting and both
sides dug in. The trenches of the Western Front materialised
and medical services, both army and voluntary, were forced to
take a longer term view and reorganise accordingly. The Eastern
Front stretched for thousands of kilometres, from Finland in the
north to Macedonia in the south; from deep into Russia in the
east to parts of the Austro–Hungarian Empire and the countries of the Balkans in the west. Following the assassination of
their crown prince, Austria–Hungary, with the support of its ally
Germany, had attacked Serbia in August 1914. Serbia successfully
repelled the Austrians in the early battles and by December 1914
had regained their capital, Belgrade. This was due in part to the
diversion of some of the Austrian army to its eastern provinces of
Galicia where the Serbs' patron Russia had invaded. Although the

Serbs had triumphed early, their army, its medical service and the Serbian population were severely depleted from fighting both the 1912–1913 Balkan Wars and the most recent battles with Austria. As the 1914–1915 winter hit they were engulfed by a devastating plague of typhus. Their need for medical assistance became urgent.

Eastern Front: Uskub, Serbia

February 1915, Winter

As a medical student, Dr Elsie Dalyell rode a motorbike and, due to her fair hair, the male students called her 'the yellow peril'. Elsie was a brilliant student, gaining first class honours on graduation from the University of Sydney in 1910 and becoming the first Australian woman to win a Beit Fellowship, one of the most prestigious postgraduate scholarships, awarded for scientific research by the Imperial College of Science and Technology in London. The fellowship took her to the Lister Institute of Preventive Medicine in London, where her research was primarily into preventive medicine, particularly the aetiology of summer diarrhoea in infants, a major cause of infant mortality at the time.

But in 1915, when she was thirty-three, Elsie put aside her research at the Lister and offered her pathology skills to unsympathetic military officials at the WO, where she was instantly turned away. Instead, she found a welcome with Lady Cornelia Wimborne's Serbian Relief Fund field hospital, and headed to the Eastern Front.

Dozens of wealthy titled British women contributed to the Allied war effort by offering their homes as military hospitals and also by funding ambulance units and mobile field hospitals, which they sometimes accompanied. Elsie was appointed as patholo-gist to the Wimborne Unit (the Serbs called it Wimbornsky) on New Year's Day 1915 and by 9 February she was headed for the Greek port of Salonica (Thessaloniki), sailing down the coasts of Portugal and Spain and through the Straits of Gibraltar. Salonica was the entry point for medical aid to Serbia, where the battles against the invading Austro–Hungarians, the rapid spread of deadly typhus and a particularly severe winter had combined to create a medical catastrophe. Unlike other types of fevers, typhus thrives in cold weather.[2]

The Great War was the first major conflict in which bacte-riology, pathology and laboratory medicine played a vital role in saving lives. Elsie and several other Australian women doctors found their pathology skills in demand. Although this was a time before the arrival of antibiotics, the swift identification of bacteria could hasten whatever treatment was available or change the nature of the treatment. Battle lines moved across vast geographic areas, causing armies to move and uproot civilian populations, particu-larly on the unstable Eastern Front. The new devastating firearms employed in battle increased the likelihood of gas gangrene, and, with the emergence of trench warfare, diseases pushed the limits of contemporary medical knowledge and demanded a response from clinical pathologists.

The need for rapid diagnosis meant that thousands of tests involving bacteria, parasites, blood and urine were conducted throughout the war. Pathologists like Elsie collected and analysed specimens for fevers, wounds and gas gangrene, diarrhoeas, and parasitic and venereal diseases. Sometimes they identified illnesses not necessarily associated with war service such as diphtheria, scarlet fever and tuberculosis, which nevertheless impacted on soldiers' health.[3] Elsie's skills in the nascent specialty of pathology were evident and the Director of the Serbian Relief Fund was delighted to greet her.

An estimated half a million Serbs fell victim to typhus in the first six months of World War I and at least 200,000 died, including 70,000 soldiers of the Serbian army. Typhus is spread by tenacious body lice, which thrive in any unhygienic situation. This made Serbia a dangerous place for any volunteer to work.[4] By early March Elsie was travelling the 250 kilometres from Salonica to Uskub (now Skopje, Macedonia) on the main railway line, which followed the valley of the Vardar River. She had arrived in Salonica 'on a blue and gold morning' and viewed Mt Olympus with its snow-covered peak in dense white cloud, surrounded by a faint bluish mist.[5]

Elsie's hospital was set up in a barracks building inside a sixth-century Turkish hilltop fort – a *kale* – looking down on the city of Uskub, which in 1915 was in Serbian Macedonia. Her unit, the second sent by the London-based Serbian Relief Fund, had forty members and included at least three male doctors, twenty nurses and a group of orderlies. Nearly all of the volunteers who joined the three Serbian Relief Fund units were women, with the only exceptions being several male surgeons and an occasional male orderly. On arrival, the unit found the *kale* in a filthy state and everyone set to work scrubbing floors and whitewashing the ancient walls. Thick walls kept both the March cold and later the summer heat out, but there was no water on tap so it had to be bailed into creosote-lined barrels and brought up from the Vardar River far below by bullock wagon. Creosote proved to be an effective water disinfectant but the nurses agreed that the taste ruined a cup of tea.[6]

Conditions were tough but Elsie found the hospital's location picturesque, with views to the foothills and mountains, clear air and 'The line of dazzling snow against a clear blue sky . . . the most wonderful sight I have yet seen'.[7]

The first Serbian Relief Fund unit, Lady Paget's Hospital, had reached Uskub in late 1914. They found a huge barracks building overflowing with more than 1500 sick and wounded and only a few doctors. All the windows were kept shut, the corridors were dark and the place smelt like a sewer. Every bit of floor space was packed with patients lying on shared mattresses and wearing dirty clothes or uniforms infested with lice. Immediately after Elsie Dalyell and English doctor Eric Bellingham-Smith arrived in the town, many members of the unit's staff, including Lady Paget, became very ill with typhus themselves. The number of patients had grown to around 2000 and they were scattered across several buildings with wounded soldiers, both newly treated and untreated, mixed in with the typhus cases. Sanitary arrangements remained almost non-existent. Elsie wrote home:

> Here there is a queer fantastic existence that doesn't seem quite real at any time . . . I don't know how to tell it all. Nothing here is orderly or regular or usual, and since I left England the constant feeling has been that of living poised on one foot and ready for instant flight . . . one is prepared for anything at any time.[8]

In the first weeks, there were terrible days when as many as 300 patients died: Serbian soldiers, Austrian prisoners of war and civilians. The Serbian funeral dirge was heard repeatedly and the traditional bell-ringing had to be suspended for fear that the bells would ring all day. The two doctors, the unit's engineer and staff hastily reorganised the patients, trying to separate the surgical cases from infectious cases.[9] Sometimes this was impossible when wounded soldiers had also become infected with typhus. Hundreds of bales and crates were unpacked in the newly cleaned spaces, the beds set up and a small but sunny room found for Elsie's lab.

Another English doctor, Dr Barrington-Ward, arrived and took charge of the surgical cases in one of the buildings while Elsie and Bellingham-Smith managed the fever hospital in the *kale*. Women and children also began to arrive and Elsie's pathology tests found that many were suffering from tuberculosis as well as being infected with typhus. She often felt that she needed the strength of ten to get through a day's work. Elsie had, however, been given £125 for laboratory equipment and was glad of her new microscope and autoclave.

The regimen that Elsie, the other doctors and the nurses set in place reduced the death rate from typhus and other infectious diseases to minimal levels, despite the hospital being understaffed from February to the end of July 1915. The work was hard, requiring hundreds of samples taken from patients, but Elsie found it 'full of interest'.[10] In her small laboratory she studied patients' test samples to diagnose typhus and its common complication diphtheria, and to differentiate between dysentery, malaria and other enteric fevers.[11] During her time at Uskub, Elsie wrote about her work to Professor David Welsh, who had been Head of Pathology at the University of Sydney during her medical studies. He afterwards said:

No disease has proved so deadly to doctors and nurses as typhus, and those who went to the relief of Serbia, when it was a hotbed of the infection, were exposed to as great a risk as if they were in the firing line.[12]

Elsie Dalyell generously attributed her survival, and that of the other medical staff, to the influence and application of their splendid nurses. The doctors had introduced hygienic waste disposal and strict protocols regarding clothing and disinfection to protect them from the lice. 'To prevent lice getting into underwear it was necessary to improvise suitable garments – not such an easy matter, since the necessary tailoring was not to be had.'[13] One-piece suits with attached feet were devised that buttoned at the neck and were worn with a close white cap, a face mask, boots or sandals with socks, and rubber gloves that had been boiled. It was compulsory for all staff to wear this garment at all times on the wards.

Living conditions were basic. Elsie's room had previously been occupied by a doctor suffering from typhus and contained a bed, a packing crate with tin jug and basin, her travelling trunk and a canvas chair. Fortunately she possessed an exceptional sense of humour. On first arriving at the *kale* at 9 pm, Elsie had

> an astounding collection of culture media, bundles of laundry, bedroom jugs . . . and other properties . . . [on] an unusual ramshackle native conveyance, and as we came through the old Turkish graveyard a wheel came off, and I came out, and all my bundles too . . . so I arrived nearly ill with laughter.[14]

The doctors hoped to create a sitting room for the staff when enough packing crates came to hand. As spring arrived, Elsie loved the appearance of cerulean cornflowers and 'the huge opium poppies . . . in white fields that look like still lakes'.[15] More staff arrived at the end of July and Elsie and her two male colleagues were recalled to England.

Eleven weeks later, on 15 October, Uskub was overrun by Bulgarian army units. Austro–Hungarian and German units had invaded Serbia from the north on 6 October and Bulgaria followed suit from the south-east. Bulgaria and Serbia were long-time foes and, encouraged by the promise of gaining territory, Bulgaria had joined the Central Powers in September 1915 and mobilised its army. The staff of the hospital units in Uskub insisted on remaining with their patients and became prisoners of war of the Bulgarians.

London, England

April 1915, Spring

Like Elsie, Dr Grace Cordingley was a graduate of both Sydney Girls High School and the University of Sydney but Grace's initial degree was in Arts. In 1907 she decided to study medicine and, using her Arts qualification as a foundation, moved with her mother to London, completing her medical degree at the London School of Medicine for Women (LSMW) in 1913.[16] The LSMW had been opened by Dr Elizabeth Garrett Anderson in 1874 in response to the almost universal opposition to educating women in medicine and to providing them with clinical experience. At the start of the war, more than half of the approximately 1000 registered women doctors in Britain had been trained at the LSMW.[17] Grace had returned home to Sydney in early 1914 but twelve months later the war brought her back to England to work in the rapidly growing area of pathology. On 24 March 1915, she boarded the RMS *Mongolia* in Sydney for her two-month sea voyage.

Arriving in London, Grace found a flat in the three-storey terrace houses of Nottingham Terrace on the edge of Regent's Park. She was immediately appointed to the Royal Free Hospital as a pathologist in a brand-new building named the Helena

Block. This was meant to house out-patients, casualty, X-rays and massage and included three wards for obstetrics and gynaecology. However, before the new departments could begin, the WO requisitioned the building and it became the Royal Free Military Hospital for Officers.[18] The imposing Georgian-style hospital was situated in Gray's Inn Road, and for Grace, the short distance from both the British Museum and the British Library must have been a bonus.

At the Royal Free, Grace gathered hundreds of patient samples from the 150 wounded or sick officers. She walked between beds covered with pale green or blue silk down-filled quilts with the screens and chairs repeating the gentle colour theme. Prolonged trench warfare on the Western Front meant that, for the wounded men, quiet and mental rest were considered as important to recovery as physical rest.

Eastern Front: Montenegro

April 1915, Spring

Famine, cold and war are the best allies of typhus and by April 1915 it was tragically obvious that the small country of Montenegro, to the west of Serbia, was suffering badly from an epidemic.[19] The country was poor and had exhausted its resources fighting the 1912–1913 Balkan Wars in order to free itself from Ottoman rule. Even before August 1914, Montenegro's government was struggling to feed its army and its people and was heavily dependent on loans from the Allied governments. The WARC responded to their plight and in February 1915 asked Dr Isabel Ormiston, who was still working in a field hospital in Belgium, to make her way to Montenegro to assess the medical situation.

Isabel, again in the company of her colleague Matron Monica Patton-Bethune, departed London's Victoria Station on 23 April 1915, most likely headed for the port of Folkestone.[20] The station was a scene of frenetic activity with soldiers both departing for and arriving from the frontline in France. Departing soldiers carried their belongings in long duffle bags and often clutched small bunches of flowers from family or well-wishers. Soldiers returning on leave – only three days in 1915 – were often very dirty, their clothes caked in mud and their faces grey. Free buffets, currency exchange kiosks and buses travelling around the metropolis were provided for them at London stations.[21]

To reach Montenegro in May 1915, Isabel sailed through the Adriatic to the main Montenegrin port of Bar, and then travelled 92 kilometres north-east to the city of Podgoritza (Podgorica). When Italy, previously neutral, declared war on Austria–Hungary in late May, the Adriatic became a war zone involving boats from the fleets of both the Allies and the Central Powers. German U-boats had been using the Adriatic as a safe harbour and both sides had laid mines. Isabel soon confirmed to the WARC back in London that the people of Montenegro were in desperate need of a hospital unit equipped with anti-typhus vaccines, disinfectants and medical incinerators.[22]

Podgoritza was divided into a Turkish district of mosques and minarets and a Christian district, which Isabel thought was the poorer. Leaders in the old Turkish part of town took full advantage of Isabel's freedom as a British woman and asked her to attend to the sequestered women of the harems who never left their own quarters. She was also invited to attend a service in the mosque – the only woman – and escorted up to the balcony of the minaret to admire the view.[23] When some nurses and a dispenser arrived ahead of the hospital being sent by the WARC, Isabel and

Monica were able to set up a military hospital with fifty patients, a huge out-patients' department and a small isolation ward with six typhus patients. Isabel worked with a local Turkish doctor who was attempting to care for the entire civilian population of the town.

Language was a great difficulty and when the doctors had to assess a Montenegrin soldier thought to be malingering, Isabel was amused that an Australian woman and a Turk had to use an Austrian patient – a prisoner of war – to translate their questions. Many of the sick were Austrian and lack of facilities and food meant that some died in the hospital from typhus, typhoid or dysentery. The men grieved that they were facing death away from their homes without their families' knowledge of their whereabouts.

Later in May the arrival of the WARC doctors and their hospital equipment was delayed because the Adriatic route was now too perilous to attempt. Instead, they arrived at Podgoritza via the longer overland route from Salonica. The port of Salonica in Greece was an anomaly in that, for the first two years of the war while headed by their king, Constantine, the country was officially neutral. Salonica had been wrested from the Turks by Greece as a result of the 1912–1913 Balkan Wars and was strategically important to the Allied armies as the main southern entrance to the Balkan Peninsula and to the Eastern Front. It was not until July 1917 that Greece declared its allegiance to the Allies.

Greece allowed the British and French armies to land their troops in the port from early 1915, and Salonica had become a vast, bustling settlement of soldiers, nurses, cars, trucks, horses, equipment, tents and military hospitals. Its street-side cafes were the great meeting places of the armies, the most famous being Floccas in Venizelos Street with dozens of little tables and hundreds of chairs. French, British, Serbian, Albanian, and Russian Kossack regiments as well as colonial soldiers such as Annamites, Senegalese, Madagascans and Indians all had their favourite places along the city's streets.[24] Later in 1917, Australian Dr Agnes Bennett wrote that on a visit to Salonica from her hospital in the north at Ostrovo, northern Macedonia, she enjoyed an excellent meal of risotto followed by Turkish coffee but that the British officers stuck with their roast beef, which she suspected was horsemeat. Salonica was unfortunately low-lying and swampy and one of Europe's worst areas for malaria. Everyone stationed there constantly battled against being bitten by pernicious mosquitoes. But for four years it was a vital access point to the Balkans for the Allied armies.

The WARC unit that Isabel had requested finally arrived in mid-June 1915. Dr Gerard Carre was in charge, accompanied by Australian Dr Lillias Hamilton and twenty more nursing staff. They were able to bring the medical equipment but could transport only some of the supplies needed for their 200-bed hospital.[25] Isabel would doubtless have found Lillias Hamilton a fascinating and possibly challenging colleague. Born in New South Wales and educated in Britain, 57-year-old Lillias was unconventional in dress and manner and a relentless campaigner for social reform for women.[26] Extraordinarily intrepid, she had established a successful medical practice in Calcutta in India and been the physician to the court of the Amir of Afghanistan in Kabul for three years – all before the turn of the century.

The staff struggled with inadequate medical supplies from the start. The stores brought from London had reached the town of Ipek (now Péc, in Kosovo) but transport was so lacking that only small quantities of drugs and bandages ever arrived in Podgoritza, which was more than 220 kilometres away. Their frustration was exacerbated by the frequent days in July and August when the temperature soared above 40°C. And soon the war caught up with them. The Austro–Hungarian offensive into Serbia had begun in October. The army and thousands of civilians retreated in appalling conditions through Albania and Montenegro to the Adriatic coast as the Austro–Hungarian army advanced. The pursuing army entered Montenegro on 5 January 1916 and by 11 January the then capital, Cetinje, 36 kilometres away, had fallen.

Isabel had entered Montenegro through the port of Bar back in May but it was now blockaded by the Austro–Hungarian navy. In early November she set out instead in the opposite direction, on a 600-kilometre trip south to the port of Salonica and, hopefully, onto a boat back to England. This meant travelling through parts of the majestic Dinaric Alps, a mountain chain spanning multiple countries where winters were harsh and snow could begin falling in late October. It also meant that Isabel had to travel at least part of the way by a sure-footed mule or mountain pony.

The party consisted of Isabel, an elderly Montenegrin colonel, his soldier servant, an interpreter and a local mountain guide as well as two pony boys. Everyone but Isabel wore the traditional clothing of the area, wide trousers with thick woollen leggings and heavy handwoven shawls for warmth.[27] The goal for the first three days was to reach Ipek, 220 kilometres away, where the WARC's precious hospital supplies had languished. The first day was taken up with eleven hours of slow motoring, but on the second day everyone mounted ponies and rode steadily for eight hours. On day three, Isabel rose in the dim morning light at 5 am to ride in drizzling rain up to a height of 8000 feet (almost 2500 metres)[28] and then make an even slower journey back down the other side. The rain produced roaring torrents as they followed the narrow, slick track along a gorge, barely able to see the sides for the heavy spray. After fifteen jarring hours, the group finally reached Ipek at 8 pm, and were thankful to find a good dinner.

The town of Ipek sits at the foot of the impressive 8839 feet (almost 2700 metres) Mt Bjeshket e Nemuna ('accursed mountain') and a day of rest was needed by everyone. Travel on the fifth day began in a horse buggy but then it was back in the saddle on ponies; they reached Metrovitza (now Mitrovicë in Kosovo) in the evening. Two more days of travel by train, including passing through Uskub where Elsie Dalyell had been several months earlier, finally brought the little party to Salonica. The trip had taken seven days and they had covered almost 700 kilometres. Isabel waited there for Monica to arrive and they travelled on to Alexandria for recuperative leave before returning to WARC headquarters in London and reassignment.[29] Later in the war years, Monica Pattone-Bethune became the Matron of the Swedish War Hospital in central London. The remaining members of the Montenegrin WARC unit, including Lillias Hamilton, undoubtedly also departed but no information of their journey is available.

Cairo, Egypt

May 1915, Spring
Agnes Bennett was born on Sydney's north shore and from a young age her bright and enquiring mind was evident. She was awarded a State Scholarship to Sydney University in 1889, the first year they were offered to girls. She thought, 'It was a wonderful day for me and beyond my wildest dreams.'[30] A very clever young woman, she was also the first woman to achieve an honours science degree at Sydney University, but no one would employ her. So she borrowed

the money to complete her medical degree at Edinburgh's College of Medicine for Women. It took her years to repay the money but this inner strength and perseverance carried her right into the heart of World War I military medicine.

Pursuing her desire to run her own private medical practice, Agnes moved to Wellington in New Zealand in 1905. She developed a large practice in the centre of the capital, becoming financially secure and gaining a sound professional reputation.[31] When three of her brothers enlisted in the Australian Imperial Force (AIF), she decided that she definitely wanted to contribute to the war effort.

When Agnes tried to enlist in Wellington, New Zealand, in early 1915, she was forty-one years old, had two medical degrees and ten years of medical experience but the New Zealand Army Medical Corps (NZAMC) was not interested in enlisting women. She brushed this off and wrote to the French Red Cross. They snapped up her offer of service immediately and asked her to report in Paris as soon as she could.

She boarded the RMS *Morea* in Sydney in mid-April 1915 taking her medical bag and paying her fare to France.[32] In the ship's hold were Red Cross parcels, medicine and wool bound for England. A week later the SS *Orontes* left Melbourne for London with twenty male doctors on board. Many had just completed their five-year medical degrees and had very little clinical experience but were nevertheless accepted for enlistment with the RAMC.[33]

Most steamships on the Sydney to Alexandria route travelled at about 25 kilometres an hour and the trip took about five weeks, calling in at the ports of Colombo and Aden. Colombo was impressively exotic, with hundreds of tiny catamaran fishing boats loaded down with bananas, pineapples and coconuts jockeying for position alongside Agnes' ship to sell their fruit, and fishermen diving for silver coins.[34] When allowed on board, the traders brought newspapers, postcards, beads and highly competitive gaiety. Less enjoyable was the terrible heat that greeted the passengers for the six-day trip through the Red Sea. Agnes enjoyed the boat's holiday atmosphere and the company of ten keen young doctors. A small company of the very new Australian Flying Corps (AFC) were on board and they enthusiastically entered into games, sports and general roughhousing.

One of the four new pilots on board with the AFC personnel had just qualified as a doctor at the University of Melbourne. Lieutenant George Merz was a final-year colleague of Dr Vera Scantlebury and Dr Rachel Champion, who would later join the war effort in a London military hospital. He took part in the AFC's first operational flights in Mesopotamia (Iraq) in late May 1915 but he was also Australia's first air-war casualty. George was killed by enemy forces on 30 July 1915 after he was forced to land his malfunctioning Caudron plane on a flight to Basra. He was twenty-three and his squadron had been in action for just eight weeks.

With no radio news, Agnes assumed that the war was progressing well for the Allies. But from Aden onwards, rumours began to circulate about heavy casualties. At the end of the 3000-kilometre trip from the Gulf of Aden, the *Morea* neared Port Said through the Suez Canal, and Agnes could see the army camps along the banks, including regiments of the Australian Light Horse. Army officers rowed out from the banks to enquire urgently whether there were newspapers on board.[35] Agnes had left New Zealand with many requests from her patients to check on the welfare and whereabouts of their 'boys' and she was also concerned for her brother, Bob. She called out to soldiers on the shore to enquire of the war's progress but they were reticent. On arrival at the port, the evidence of the toll from the Dardanelles campaign was clear. Australian and New Zealand soldiers were being unloaded onto Port Said's docks from the hospital ship the *Guilford Castle* and their stretchers lay in the intense heat. A line of ambulances moved along the dock and, horrified, Agnes realised they were AIF wounded from the Gallipoli battlefields.

The Gallipoli campaign was devised by the British army to put the Ottoman Empire out of the war. The plan was to bombard the coastal forts, land Allied troops and sweep on to the Turkish capital Constantinople (now Istanbul). The initial attack failed disastrously and eight months of desperate fighting took place across the Gallipoli Peninsula as the Turks fiercely resisted the invasion of their homeland. Between 25 April 1915 and January 1916, 11,410 Australian and New Zealand (ANZAC) soldiers died and almost 18,000 Australians were wounded. The hospital ships took three and a half days to reach Alexandria and many of the wounded men had waited four or five days for medical attention.

Agnes hurriedly offered her services as a surgeon and was gladly accepted by Colonel Matthew Holmes, New Zealand's Director of Medical Services. He was working on the dock attempting to get the soldiers out of the sun and heat as quickly as possible.[36] Doctors, drugs and equipment were scarce in the early months as the Cairo hospitals received the wounded and sick from the peninsula. Agnes was given the honorary rank of captain and began the next morning at the No. 2 New Zealand Stationary Hospital at Pont de Koubbeh in Abbassia, Cairo. It was 19 May 1915 and the day of a major Turkish counterattack at Gallipoli. As she worked, Agnes asked each soldier if he had any news of her brother Bob until one confirmed that Bob was alive and acting as a stretcher-bearer. Her brother had carried the wounded soldier down to the beach at Gallipoli for transfer at nightfall to a lighter, which took the wounded out to the hospital ships.

The Pont de Koubbeh hospital was a large stone building with deep verandahs to keep out the sun. Typically, the hospital building was flat roofed and gave a stunning view of the distant hills, which shaded into faint mauves at sunset. Towards Cairo, mosques and minarets were outlined against the sky at dusk.[37]

Beginning with 250 beds it soon expanded to house more than 1000 patients with the addition of large marquees and hospital tents pitched on the desert sand.[38] Three weeks after Agnes' arrival, on 8 and 9 June, 1047 patients arrived from the hospital ships.[39] The strain on the staff was enormous and the work relentless as wounded and sick soldiers poured in, many arriving with their first field dressing from the Gallipoli fighting still in place. Sepsis can lead to gas gangrene and then to amputation, which was heartbreaking work for surgeons like Agnes. Many of the soldiers she treated also suffered from typhoid or dysentery.

After four months at Pont de Koubbeh, Agnes moved to the Choubra Infectious Diseases Hospital for the British. She was shocked to discover that the Egyptian orderlies treated all china equipment alike and stored the bedpans with the kitchen china. Agnes quickly began a training program, with hygiene in the wards as a central tenet.[40] She wrote from Choubra to the New Zealand newspapers and to influential women friends to say that when the wounded and sick 'boys' arrived from the hospital ships, only a small hospital kit was available for each. Amenities were in very short supply and they needed clothing, sweets and tobacco urgently.

Agnes was popular with the nurses and they made her an honorary member of the Nurses of the Empire Club provided by the Red Cross.[41] The club was opened in a fine house and garden, where the nurses could relax, invite guests for afternoon tea and play tennis on the grass court. When there was time,

Agnes wrote from the shade of the spacious verandahs at Cairo's Grand Continental Hotel. The British had taken over the hotel's accommodation and at times during the war it was also home to Gertrude Bell and Colonel TE Lawrence, better known as Lawrence of Arabia.

When she was off duty, Agnes visited Egypt's ancient icons at Luxor and Karnak and photographed the famous buildings, ruins and sculptures. But she also liked to record people at their work – photographing water-carriers, farmers, pottery sellers and manure-carriers – and was interested in the technology of the water wheels and the different methods of obtaining water from the Nile for irrigation. She photographed Egyptian nurses and midwives and their patients wearing traditional abaya, and Armenian women who visited from their refugee camp.

London, England

July 1915, Summer
While Agnes was dealing with the fearful casualties from the Dardanelles campaign, Dr Emma Buckley departed from Sydney clutching a letter of introduction to the Lister Institute in London. The institute, established in London in 1891, researched the causes, prevention and treatment of diseases in both humans and animals and developed preventive and curative medicines such as vaccines and anti-toxins.[42] It was a prestigious place to work, its renown in line with the Pasteur Institute in Paris and the Rockefeller Institute in New York. Emma's colleague, Dr Elsie Dalyell, had been pursuing her Beit Scholarship at the Lister until the typhus epidemic in Serbia had demanded her expertise in bacteriology.

Like Grace Cordingley and Elsie Dalyell, Emma had been a student at Sydney Girls High School and a boarder at the University of Sydney's Women's College. She began her university studies in science but changed to medicine and discovered a keen lifetime interest in pathology. As she left Sydney Harbour on the SS *Osterley* on 5 May 1915, rain and gale force winds made for an anxious start. But Emma reached London safely in mid-July 1915. She found the city swarming with wounded soldiers who wore blue armbands while convalescing, as well as soldiers on leave from the front and those about to leave for France. Recruiting rallies were everywhere but the English crowds seemed less enthusiastic than those she had seen in Sydney. She thought the Londoners' 'business-as-usual attitude' made them seem almost indifferent.[43]

Wasting no time, she went straight to the Lister Institute. They were short-handed and under intense pressure for test results and vaccines for the sick and wounded.

Emma had been introduced to the Lister's Director, Dr Charles Martin, by a letter from her University of Sydney professor, Sir Thomas Anderson Stuart. As Dean of Medicine, Stuart had recruited Martin from England to teach in Sydney for a time before Martin's brilliance in scientific research led to his appointment to the Lister in London. Anderson Stuart had been a strong supporter of women students in medicine and both Emma and another of her Sydney colleagues, Dr Elizabeth Hamilton-Browne, benefited from his English connections. Before the war, the Lister Institute's work had included the development of sera for smallpox, typhoid and diphtheria, and from the beginning of hostilities they stepped up their production of tetanus anti-toxins. Their work also included the identification of the bacteria that caused the deadly gas gangrene in infected wounds.[44] Martin obviously had confidence in students educated by Anderson Stuart and Emma was awarded a one-year Jenner Research Scholarship of £150.

At first Emma was given an 'apprenticeship' for several weeks in making media for testing samples, but quickly proving herself, she then began work on developing methods for drying various sera to create an easily transportable and compact powder. This could then be dissolved in saline and be ready for testing samples wherever and whenever it was required – a much more convenient medium for the battlefields. The powders were then sent to the Mediterranean island of Lemnos where Dr Martin was testing their efficacy.

Infectious diseases were commonplace across Europe in 1914. People became ill with bacterial diseases such as cholera, typhoid, tuberculosis and typhus and with viral diseases such as influenza, measles and poliomyelitis. Diseases spread by parasites, lice and mites, such as malaria and typhus, flourished in wartime conditions. Microbes and the diseases they caused were enemies as treacherous as the Germans.[45] Emma's pathology work from July 1915 to later in 1916 included making typhoid, paratyphoid and cholera vaccines and testing water supplies. She collected samples from the soldiers at the King George Military Hospital, England's largest with around 1900 beds. Back in the laboratory she then tested blood and urine samples and throat swabs for venereal disease and illnesses like diphtheria, tuberculosis and dysentery.

In her first six or seven months at the Lister, Emma was supervised by bacteriologist Sir William Penfold, who was treating many Australian soldiers invalided to the King George from Gallipoli with dysentery infections. Penfold had been tasked by the RAMC to produce an anti-typhoid vaccine and in 1916 was appointed as the Director of the new Commonwealth Serum Laboratories back in Australia.

Emma's work at the Lister came to an end later in 1916 and she was appointed to the Endell Street Military Hospital in London's Covent Garden district, commonly known as 'the suffrage hospital'. The Endell Street Military Hospital and the WHC were created by doctors Flora Murray and Louisa Garrett Anderson.[46] Both were members of the Women's Social and Political Union (WPSU), a militant suffrage organisation begun by feminists Emmeline and Christabel Pankhurst. Flora and Louisa had taken immediate and full advantage of the administrative shambles of medical organisation at the beginning of the war. As experienced suffrage campaigners, they were well aware that women doctors offering to enlist would be rejected. They bypassed English officialdom and called on the French Embassy just eight days after war had been declared, where a combination of the women's rusty French and the embassy's strong desire to acquire urgently needed medical supplies and equipment paved the way for them to establish a military hospital in France.[47] Given the antipathy with which both the WO and RAMC greeted offers of help from women doctors and the negative response of the French government to their own women medicos, this was surprising. Flora Murray believed that the French may simply not have understood that the women meant to staff the hospital themselves.[48]

The two doctors raised money, designed WHC uniforms for doctors and orderlies, recruited eighteen other staff, and bought copious supplies and transported it all to Paris in four weeks, from mid-August to mid-September 1914. With WPSU badges pinned to their uniforms, they opened their first military hospital in the brand-new hastily converted Hotel Claridge on 22 September 1914.[49] By 6 November they had opened a second hospital in the Chateau Mauricien at Wimereux near Boulogne and had 165 beds in the two hospitals. At Wimereux, wounded soldiers came directly from the frontline, covered in mud and often wet to the waist and 'the rate of mortality was lamentably high'.[50]

The task was intimidating and the risks great, but Louisa and Flora were audacious, determined and organised. Flora believed that working for a militant suffrage movement before the war had developed the discipline and extraordinary stamina required to achieve this breakthrough for women doctors and the surgical skills they rapidly needed to acquire. Five months were sufficient to demonstrate their capacity for both management and medicine.

Sir Alfred Keogh, Director General of British Army Medical Services, was so impressed when he heard about their work at their Paris hospital that he immediately offered the vast eighteenth-century St Giles Workhouse in Covent Garden for the establishment of a large military hospital. Unfortunately, even encouragement from the highest level of the WO did not readily filter down to the RAMC and in the three months it took to open the hospital, the Officers Commanding (OCs) withstood hostility and obstruction. Despite this, the Endell Street Military Hospital was accredited by the WO and was the only military hospital run by women within the British army during World War I.[51]

The St Giles Workhouse was said to be the very one described by Charles Dickens in *Oliver Twist* and sat in the middle of the swarming streets of Soho and Drury Lane. Small exercise yards were still in place – labelled 'Old Males', 'Young Males', 'Old Females' and 'Young Females' – and the mortuary had slate pigeonholes large enough to take coffins. The building was five storeys high and required lifts big enough to hold stretchers and their bearers to be fitted. Electricity had to be installed, bathrooms and wardrooms created on every floor, and rooms converted to operating theatres, an X-ray facility, laboratories, dispensaries and storerooms.[52] There was also a mortuary and an incinerator, which produced an appalling smell when amputated limbs were burnt.

Emma Buckley said that the hospital had been 'founded on broken glass',[53] referring to the staunch suffrage history of its founders, Dr Louisa Garrett Anderson and Dr Flora Murray. With the exception of a small RAMC unit, the 180 staff at the Endell Street Military Hospital were female – doctors, nurses, orderlies and Voluntary Aid Detachments (VADs). Emma did not agree with the OCs' political views but thought the hospital was very well run and hoped to be appointed as its registrar. But after only two or three months she was sent to the laboratory at the King George Military Hospital to continue work on a particular strain of dysentery.

Croydon, England

July 1915, Summer

Elsie Dalyell also arrived back in London in July 1915, returning from her pathology work in Serbia, and she was immediately employed at Addington Park Military Hospital, Croydon. Over decades, the mansion house had previously been home to six Archbishops of Canterbury. It initially held 150 beds but temporary wards for 200 more were soon added. During the war the 350-bed hospital specialised in the convalescence of patients with an acute infectious enteric disease such as typhoid, paratyphoid and dysentery. Elsie's laboratory, searching for their elusive aetiology, carried out tests to identify infection carriers at other London military hospitals, who were then immediately transferred to Addington Park.

Soldiers recovering from septicaemia, a dangerous infection of the blood stream, were also treated at the hospital. The infection generally resulted from wounds but could also be the result of simple scratches and mosquito bites. Patients mostly stayed for six to eight weeks and 150 of the beds were set aside for Australian soldiers, who in 1915 most commonly were suffering from dysentery contracted at Gallipoli.

Western Front: Paris, France

July 1915, Summer

While Elsie Dalyell was working as a pathologist at Addington Park, across the English Channel in Paris, Dr Helen Sexton was opening her hospital. The Hôpital Australien de Paris began in July 1915 with twenty-one beds and was given French military status as a branch of their army's Val de Grâce Military Hospital.[54] The French Red Cross provided the location: a spacious villa in the 16th arrondissement of Paris at Auteuil, just across the Rue du Docteur Blanche from the beautiful Parisian racecourse, which became home to an extensive American Red Cross Hospital in 1918. Helen was appointed *médecin majeur* by the French military.[55]

Her '*les petits blessés*', wounded French soldiers, were moved between different hospitals, sometimes five or six times, according to the nature and severity of their wounds, complications and where the hospital beds were available.[56] Most commonly patients were moved between Helen's Hôpital and the Lycée Buffon, a large high school converted to the Buffon Military Hospital, 4 kilometres away across the river Seine.

Always interested in more than just the immediate medical problems of her patients, and with a good grasp of the French language, Helen recorded each patient's war service including the battle where the wound had occurred. These notes, still surviving, are a rare window into the daily life of a woman surgeon handling whatever cases arrived. The complexity and challenges of World War I military medicine are very clear in her case notes. Julien Godot was one of her first patients. He was admitted on 19 July 1915 with a shrapnel wound that had penetrated his sacrum joint at the base of his spine and was causing paralysis in his right leg and the retention of urine. He was twenty-two years old and had already been wounded three times. Helen also devoted an entire page to the story of a French colonial soldier from Tunisia. He arrived twelve days after Julien with shrapnel wounds to his thigh from a battle near Ypres in late April. Unable to stand, he had propelled himself backwards on his elbows for 4 kilometres searching for help. Dehydrated and extremely thirsty, he crawled underneath a cow hoping to steal a little milk. Instead, the cow provided only a swift kick to his head. Eventually he was found by a British field ambulance team.

Another patient, Edouard Deracuias, had contracted typhoid after six months in the Allied trenches near Verdun and been admitted to Buffon in the first week of May 1915. On 31 July he was transferred to Helen's care with post-typhoid alveolar periostitis. This is a complication from typhoid that causes very severe pain in the jaw and Helen immediately incised and removed all of the dead bone and affected teeth. Jean Badaud, admitted in early November, required further surgery to his leg wounds and Helen painstakingly removed shreds of his uniform and the half of a bomb screw that remained embedded in his leg. Unfortunately an X-ray machine was not available on that day and her surgical explorations took longer and were more tenuous. She recorded injuries from automobile accidents, fractures, gangrene, pneumonia, tuberculosis, syphilis, frostbite, aching teeth and abscesses. The war demanded a comprehensive set of medical skills at a time when doctors were generalists and medical specialisation was only beginning to grow.

The Hôpital Australien closed on 10 December 1915 and Helen was then invited to work as an Assistant Surgeon at Val de Grâce, which specialised in the meticulous facial reconstruction surgery that horribly wounded soldiers required. After the war, the French Government awarded her the Gold Médaille de la Reconnaissance Française. This honour is reserved for those who, without legal or military obligation, came to the aid of the injured or act with exceptional dedication in the presence of the enemy.[57] It is not known how long Helen remained at Val de Grâce but she returned home to Melbourne in April 1916.

Western Front: Calais, France

September 1915, Autumn
In the first half of 1915, a new University of Sydney graduate, Dr Katie Ardill, was considering how best to be useful to the war effort. Katie was completing her residency at Sydney's Royal Prince Alfred Hospital when the war erupted and, over the following months, she determined to go to England to offer her skills. Her father, George, told her she was not to go and refused to help her with the boat fare. The AAMC had also declined her offer to enlist. Undaunted by either, Katie borrowed the one-way fare, which was either £60–£70 for first class or £35–£40 for second class, and sailed from Sydney on 26 June 1915.[58] She travelled on the RMS *Medina*, a handsome boat, its funnels decorated with royal blue and gold stripes from an earlier trip by British royalty

from London to India. Katie's father was justified in his concern. Although Katie reached England safely, the *Medina* was later sunk off the English coast near Devon by a German U-boat torpedo in 1917.

Katie carried a letter to Sir George Reid, former Australian Prime Minister and Australia's first High Commissioner to London. He sent her to Sir Frederick Treves, a surgeon associated with the British Red Cross and famous for his work with Joseph Merrick, known by the pitiless term 'the elephant man'. Surprised at first by her insistence on volunteering, Treves initially refused but finally helped her to join the British Red Cross No. 2 Anglo–Belgian Military Hospital for Belgian soldiers.[59] By September 1915, she was at work in the hospital a few blocks from the French port of Calais and its dockside train station. Calais, where the channel is at its narrowest, was a major, hectic access point for soldiers and supplies throughout the war and on clear days Katie could see the white cliffs of Dover from the port.

The 166-bed hospital was primarily for typhoid and infectious diseases patients and Katie was the only female medical officer. Her arrival caused consternation and initially the medical staff appeared to be terrified by the idea of a woman doctor.[60] Katie's patients wore the distinctive blue uniform and red tie that military authorities required all recovering soldiers to wear in hospital and out in public. The uniform became known popularly as 'hospital blues' and helped with hospital hygiene because soldiers usually arrived in their dirty, muddy infested uniforms and greatcoats, both requiring disinfection or disposal. Hospital blues were easily washed but their one-size-fits-all and pocket-less design was not always appreciated by patients.

Calais was under martial law when Katie arrived, with all lights out at 8 pm. She worked in the wooden hut wards built around an old house, the only luxury being the provision of electric light. But the sunlight poured in during summer, with almost every bed having a window, and the wards were decorated with flags and flowers. A similar sparsely furnished hut with walls pasted with pictures cut from newspapers and maps served as a staff common-room for the Belgian doctor in charge, three medical officers, the nurses and orderlies.[61] Katie worked at the hospital for six months until she was redeployed to Middlesex in England in March 1916.

London, England

Early 1915, Winter
When Queenslander Mabel Murray-Prior heard that Britain was at war, she was visiting Hong Kong but she travelled on to London in 1915 to offer her services. Mabel had completed three years of the medical course at the University of Sydney but, like Isabel Ormiston and Grace Cordingley, had begun her studies with a first year in the Arts Faculty. She began medicine with Isabel, Grace and also Elsie Dalyell but, as with many of her contemporaries, male and female, she took subjects over more years than the minimum five. Mabel was from Maroon in the picturesque hinterland of the area now known as the Gold Coast in southern Queensland and her family was at the centre of Queensland's social and political life. However, her university studies and future were disrupted when her mother died in 1901, when Mabel was nineteen, and her father the following year in 1902.

In February 1915 the WO proposed that volunteers could help at military hospitals. These had previously been staffed exclusively by army nurses and male orderlies from the RAMC. A group known as Voluntary Aid Detachments (VADs) – or as the soldiers called them, 'Very Adorable Darlings' – had been set up in 1911 and by 1914 there were 40,000 volunteers in 1800 detachments. Initially they were trained to provide meals for soldiers at train stations and to care for the wounded briefly during transfers but in 1912 a small number went away to the Balkan Wars – the conflict where Dr Laura Forster had served. The demand for medical services from the start of World War I meant their role broadened rapidly and from February 1915 they worked in hospitals as nursing assistants, ambulance drivers and administration; in fact anything and everything.[62] Mabel served as a VAD throughout 1915 and then decided to complete her medical degree so that she could contribute to the war as a doctor.

One of the organisations that attracted women doctors and nurses across the Empire was the SWH. Over the course of World War I, six Australian women doctors served with the SWH in France, Serbia, Galicia and Russia. In Edinburgh in July 1914, Dr Elsie Inglis, a Scottish suffragist, had devised a radical plan for mobile hospital units – fully staffed by women – to support the British Expeditionary Forces' medical units. Just as all offers of service by women doctors were denied, her attempt to enlist with the RAMC was rejected with peremptory disregard by the imperial authorities.

Elsie then extended the offer of SWH units to other Allied governments. Faced with unprecedented losses, huge numbers of injured servicemen and shortages of medical personnel, the governments of Belgium, Russia, France and Serbia all responded enthusiastically. British women did not have the vote in 1914 but had developed strong suffrage groups and networks. By mobilising the National Union of Women's Suffrage Societies (NUWSS),

Dr Elsie Inglis and its president, Millicent Fawcett, had a ready network of women to support them both locally and internationally. Through the course of the war, the NUWSS organised fourteen SWH mobile hospitals to operate in proximity to the battlefields, as well as a base hospital at Royaumont Abbey near Asnières-sur-Oise, 30 kilometres north of Paris. It took just three months from Dr Inglis' original plan for the first unit to travel to Calais in France.[63]

The SWH units operating during the period of 1914–1919 served at: Calais, Royaumont, Troyes, Sallanches and Corsica in France; Kragujevac, Valjevo, Mladanovatz (Mladenovac) and Lazarovatz (Lazarevac) in Serbia; Salonica in Greece; Ostrovo in Macedonia;[64] Galicia; and Russia.

Some units were set up in existing premises, such as the abbey at Royaumont near Asnières-sur-Oise, which operated from 1915 to 1919. Others were in large canvas tents, such as the America Unit with the Third Serbian Army at Ostrovo, in northern Macedonia. The field hospital units moved according to requests from Allied armies or followed the war fronts to be on hand when casualties poured in.[65] In addition, the NUWSS also sent equipped hospital corps, such as the Millicent Fawcett Hospitals, to countries such as Russia to work with the civilian casualties and refugees of war.[66] Although the intention in Russia and Galicia was to alleviate the suffering of civilians, the maelstrom of war often meant they were caring for wounded soldiers as well.

The SWH was administered from Edinburgh and London; their doctors performed surgery, managed a wide range of illnesses and provided pathology, pharmacy and X-ray services. They also oversaw all the sanitary arrangements in the camps and quickly learned the importance of good drainage, trenches and the constant redigging of latrines as well as keeping records of the latrines' previous whereabouts. Each unit included nurses, women orderlies and others who drove the ambulances, maintained motor vehicles, cooked, laundered and managed the supplies and some of the endless paperwork. It was a professional entity, run along the same lines as the military. Chief medical officers were in charge of each unit and reported to the army command wherever they were situated as well as to the SWH headquarters in Edinburgh. Most of the staff were paid for their work and women from all classes were recruited, working at all levels.

The SWH designed their own uniform of light grey wool with tartan trim and it was to be worn at all times. Like all the women's voluntary organisations during the war, a great deal of thought was given to the design of uniforms. For the first time, women were wearing military-style clothing that had previously been the preserve of men.[67] New roles meant new dress codes, both for practicality and to reflect the military nature of their organisations, and provided a public statement of the commitment of women to war service. Women in uniform also attracted attention. The SWH units followed the military model with discipline, codes of conduct and curfews; all were considered essential and enforced.

Eastern Front: Serbia

September 1915, Autumn
Dr Laura Fowler Hope and her husband, Dr Charles Hope, both from Adelaide, were the first Australian doctors to join the SWH. Strongly motivated by Baptist Christian values, Laura had written enthusiastically to her father in May 1898: 'I want to be as much use in the world as I can.'[68]

Born in Adelaide, South Australia, in 1868, she had already shown her determination and intellectual ability as the first woman to enrol in medicine at the University of Adelaide in South Australia in 1887. There was opposition as she was only eighteen years of age but she had the support of Professor Archie Watson, who the medical students called 'proffie'. She topped the results list in her first year, won the coveted Elder Prize for physiology in her final year and became the first South Australian woman to qualify as a medical doctor in 1891, also becoming a member of the British Medical Association (BMA). Laura was raised in Adelaide's small upper class in a successful entrepreneurial family and regarded the British Empire with great patriotism, as was common for most Australians of her class at the time.

After practising for a year at the Adelaide Children's Hospital, she married Dr Charles Hope in 1893. Seeking adventure and service, the Hopes set off overseas, travelling to Britain and to East Bengal in northern India to work as mission doctors.[69] Remaining childless, they were free to devote their lives to their healing work in India, which spanned forty years, with an interruption when they decided in September 1915 to sail to London to join the SWH. Perhaps what finally persuaded 47-year-old Laura, and Charles, aged fifty-six, to plunge into war service was that Laura's nephew had enlisted, been wounded and was recuperating in a London hospital.[70] Their time with the SWH would prove to be tumultuous.

Laura wrote to her brother Jim before leaving London, stating that hundreds were dying every day from typhus in Serbia and that she and Charles had much experience of the disease in Bengal and could be of service. Leaving England in early October, their ship passed through a Mediterranean Sea crawling with German destroyers, but they arrived safely at Salonica after a week's sailing.[71] Laura and Charles were posted to different SWH units. Responding to the typhus epidemic, three SWH units had been set up along a line stretching approximately 100 kilometres from Mladanovatz (Mladenovac, Serbia) to the east, through Lazarovatz (Lazarevac, Serbia) to Valjevo in the west – all three were south of Serbia's capital, Belgrade. Laura's unit was in Mladanovatz, a 300-bed hospital established in July 1915 and headed by Scot Dr Beatrice McGregor.

Laura's 560-kilometre train trip from Salonica to Mladanovatz was broken at Nish (Niš), where the new hospital staff stayed at the British High Commission's rest house for Red Cross workers, established by Sir Ralph Paget. Paget was an English diplomat in Serbia, given the role by the British government to oversee the voluntary units there during the war. His wife, Lady Paget, was still in Uskub running her hospital, where Dr Elsie Dalyell had worked three months previously. Laura arrived at Mladanovatz on 10 October and met the SWH founder Dr Elsie Inglis, who liked to meet new arrivals personally. This was Laura's first meeting with the small, energetic Scottish doctor but there was no time for settling in. She started immediately, assisting doctors Chesney and McGregor as they worked frantically to cope with the huge backlog of operations and the terrible presence of gas gangrene in the wounds.

Laura's husband, Charles, had been assigned to Dr Alice Hutchinson's unit at Valjevo, about 100 kilometres west of Mladanovatz. Earlier in 1915, Valjevo had been stricken with a typhus epidemic following the occupation and subsequent retreat of the Austrian army. The upheaval and battles had left behind a terrible medical situation and the Hutchinson unit had been in place since June.[72] They had relieved the women who had been running a hospital set up by the British Serbian Relief Fund, battling the typhus outbreak in appalling conditions. Doctors and nurses were at great risk and twenty-one doctors died during that terrible spring, causing a dire shortage of medical personnel. In early October 1915, with autumn fading into winter, the Germans and Austrians attacked and Serbia's capital, Belgrade, fell on 8 October.[73] Laura and Charles had arrived at the worst possible time.

The Valjevo camp, where Charles began working, had been established on a hill with a view over the town and consisted of forty wooden-floored tents with capacity for 500 patients. It would have been a beautiful site in the springtime with wild flowers carpeting the hills, but in summer everyone had battled with the swarms of flies. The hospital sat adjacent to a railway line, which proved to be very useful. Almost immediately after Charles' arrival, the hospital was evacuated from the hillside by train in an attempt to escape capture by a rapidly advancing enemy.[74]

As she worked in the operating theatre at Mladanovatz, Laura could also hear the booming guns of an approaching army. The town was in the path of the advancing enemy so on 12 October her unit was hastily evacuated to Kragujevac, 17 kilometres south-west of Mladanovatz.

On arrival, she accompanied Dr Inglis to inspect some artillery sheds as a possible site for the wards of their next hospital, with staff to be accommodated in tents. On the hospital's first day Laura observed the surgical procedures required for an amputation and worked with Dr Inglis on the following day, admitting thirty wounded. By the end of their first week, Laura's ward had received 180 patients. For three of those days she was too busy and too weary to walk back to her tent and just lay down to sleep in the ward's dressing room. The hospital occupied two sheds and on some days more than 150 patients were admitted; around 1000 wounded and sick men arrived within a week.

Laura dressed wounds continuously in the packed wards where patients were allotted three men per two beds. But after thirteen non-stop days, her unit was again ordered to evacuate, and on 25 October they moved on to Kraljevo, 55 kilometres further to the south-west. The enemy was advancing rapidly and it was a terrifying time of enormous uncertainty and fear. However, they set up a dressing station in Kraljevo anyway and many patients were treated and quickly sent southwards, hopefully to safety. On the final day of October, Laura made a last-minute decision to join her husband, who was still with Dr Hutchinson's unit. Charles' unit was leaving by train for Vrinjatcha Bania (Vrnjacka Banja, Serbia), 30 kilometres southwards and to the east of where Laura's unit was, and she joined him there. The picturesque town of Vrinjatcha Bania, with its thermal spas and medieval buildings, sat along a valley between two mountain ranges but no one had time to appreciate their surroundings.[75] Laura's choice to join her husband was a critical one. Had she stayed with Dr McGregor's unit she would have joined them in the 'Great Serbian Retreat'. Hundreds of thousands of Serbians, including the remnants of their army and civilians, fled along mule tracks through the Albanian and Montenegrin mountains in freezing temperatures and snow. Dr McGregor's unit walked for seven weeks before reaching the Adriatic and eventually boarding a ship to Brindisi, in Italy, and home. But approximately 150,000 Serbian men, women and children died from hunger and cold along the way.

The Hutchinson unit set up a hospital in Vrinjatcha Bania, with the staff staying in two local villas left empty by fleeing families. The situation became even more fluid when Bulgaria joined the German–Austrian attack and invaded Serbia from the east. Although the SWH units had fled south and finally east, Serbia was now being assailed on two fronts. Wounded continued to arrive and Laura and Charles were busy in the operating theatre and dressing wounds.[76] On 6 November, the Serbian orderlies fled, and four days later the medical staff all awoke to the horrifying discovery that the Austrian army had quietly taken possession of the town during the night. Laura, Charles and the SWH unit were now all prisoners of war. There was confusion and intense anxiety as they awaited their fate but Laura emanated a deep feeling of calm derived from her strong religious faith.[77]

No definitive answer about their situation was forthcoming. The Germans wanted Dr Hutchinson's unit to work with their wounded soldiers and after three weeks everyone was put on a train to Krushevatz (Krusevac, Serbia), 45 kilometres to the east, where there was supposedly an Austrian army hospital. Winter had arrived and the trip from Vrinjatcha Bania began with an 11-kilometre walk through the snow to the nearest railway station. The town of Krushevatz had been bombed and the women were allocated an empty barracks building to open the hospital. No one was expecting their arrival and the only accommodation available was a filthy hotel.

They did not remain in Krushevatz for long. At 4 am on 4 December, Laura's party of thirty-four was packed into cattle trucks for a journey of 160 kilometres.[78] It took thirty-six jolting and sleepless hours on roads crowded with trucks and soldiers. Stopped overnight, they were given no food or lodging by their hostile German guards and after a day and a half with no food everyone was very hungry. They resorted to begging some soup from a Red Cross kitchen nearby.[79] Arriving at Semendria (Smedereva, Serbia) on the southern bank of the river Danube, they were jeered by the soldiers from a German battalion as they waited to be ferried across and put ashore on the Hungarian side. Shown into a hut full of Austrian soldiers, they all tried to get a little sleep lying on rough benches and tables or lying along the floor. The night was freezing, with the cold seeping through everything, and again they went hungry.

Previously, the American Consulate in Austria had ensured that groups of Allied prisoners were well treated, but on this occasion the arrangements failed miserably. The party was moved on to Kevevara (Kovin, Serbia), another 150 kilometres north 'on the edge of the Hungarian plain . . . that stretches to eternity'.[80] On arrival, Laura's group was housed in two unfurnished rooms with straw as their only bedding. As there had been a cholera outbreak, they were quarantined for five days and forbidden to exercise, except in a small back yard. Their CMO, Dr Alice Hutchinson, wrote: 'we developed a forgotten prowess at rounders and other games.'[81] Water had to be fetched daily from a well and everyone spent hours in the intensifying cold, scrounging for firewood. A miserable allowance of coffee, sour bread and watery soup meant that they would have starved had they not sold whatever they could from their luggage in order to buy food.[82]

As their imprisonment rolled into December, it must have felt like being in limbo, with nowhere to escape to and no news as to their future. The locals, however, were very kind to the women prisoners, smuggling food to them when they were out collecting firewood by carefully slipping small items of food into their pockets.[83] An Italian family hid eggs in the water buckets where the women went to draw water from the well. The Austrian army asked Dr Hutchinson to staff a hospital and she agreed but insisted that her staff be inoculated against cholera and paid salaries. The work never eventuated and they loathed their enforced idleness. Laura had no idea how long they would all remain captive, hungry and monotonously unoccupied, and they were told only that they would eventually be 'exchanged'. 'The monotony of life was appalling . . . each day was a lifetime, each week a century, and never a day passed but some-one felt desperate.'[84]

To counteract the boredom and keep up their spirits, they organised concerts, games and plays which, due to the cold, had to be performed inside in their cramped surrounds. On Christmas Day 1915, Dr Hutchinson ingeniously obtained a Christmas tree and the women sang carols. A local hotel prepared a Christmas dinner for them and on that day their stomachs were full. She wrote proudly:

> a body of women of all sorts and kinds has shown itself capable of standing solidly together, and of cheerfully facing physical discomforts which none of us were accustomed to.[85]

The reality was that the women still had no idea of how much longer they would be POWs.

Early in the New Year Laura learned that they were no longer regarded as POWs but were to be treated as *interned*, although the difference remained unclear. They were transferred to the care of the police, who then restricted their movements. The women were to be housed at the police station and had to pay their own expenses. Their initial optimism evaporated when they realised that their new accommodation was even more crowded than their previous rooms. Sixteen women were each packed into two small rooms and again straw was the only bedding option. Laura and Charles, however, were given a small alcove in which to sleep. On 29 January 1916, during the eleventh week of their captivity, everyone was placed on a train and moved 340 kilometres

northward to Keceskemet (Kecskemet, Hungary), a small town
near Budapest, where the women were initially housed in a hospital
for venereal diseases. Dr Hutchinson objected strongly to this
treatment and demanded better accommodation. Keceskemet,
however, had a very welcome public bath house and the women
took delight in luxuriating in its deep hot baths.[86]

Another week dragged by before they were finally sent by
train to Budapest and on to Vienna, finally reaching the Swiss
border on 8 February 1916. They were free and delirious with joy,
and the Union Jack that Dr Hutchinson had worn underneath
her clothing ever since they left Vrinjatcha Bania was waved
from the train window.[87] Greeted with much acclaim, they were
desperate for news, having heard nothing from home for four
months.[88] Travelling by train from Bern via Paris, they sailed
across the English Channel and finally arrived in London on
12 February.[89] Laura thought all of the women had shown real
courage and their OC, Alice Hutchinson, known as 'The Little
General', had been wonderfully assertive and simply splendid.
Another staff member believed that Alice's assertiveness had
resulted in her bearing the brunt of the horrible verbal abuse
that had come their way.

After their tumultuous and anxious months in Serbia and
Hungary, Laura and Charles recuperated in London for more
than a month. The SWH wanted to appoint Laura as chief
medical officer of a new unit, to be sent with the Serbian army
when they eventually returned to the field. The men who had
survived the retreat through the mountains had been evacuated to Corfu and Corsica and would eventually regroup and
attempt to regain their homeland. However, Charles, who was
fifty-six by 1917, was struggling to cope mentally and suffering
from Bright's disease and Laura felt it unwise to accept. For

their services, Laura Fowler Hope and Charles Hope were both awarded the Serbian Samaritan Cross in 1918 by the Serbian government.[90]

Cairo, Egypt

November 1915, Autumn

At around the same time the Hopes became prisoners of the Austrians, Dr Lucy Gullett left Sydney in November 1915, hoping to serve with the Red Cross in Egypt or Lemnos or perhaps the island of Malta, which was known as the 'Nurse of the Mediterranean'. Since the beginning of June, the casualty lists and honour rolls had burgeoned in Australia's newspapers and everyone's duty to the Empire was extolled. Lucy Gullett was the seventh woman to graduate from the University of Sydney Medicine Faculty (in 1900) and, like four other women doctors to serve overseas, she was a product of Sydney Girls High School. Lucy's parents were journalists and the family valued education and literature, although Lucy loved nothing more than a day at the races. She had practised in the New South Wales town of Bathurst for five years before returning to Sydney to take up a practice on the city's north shore. Lucy was thirty-nine when she decided to offer her services and she embarked on the RMS *Mongolia* in mid-November 1915. Later in the war, the *Mongolia* would suffer the same fate as Katie Ardill's ship, when it hit a mine five hours out from Bombay with some loss of life.

Arriving in Egypt around Christmas time, Lucy found work with the Red Cross in Cairo for four months, most likely in the convalescent hospitals established for recovery and rehabilitation. The No. 1 Australian General Hospital had set up two convalescent hospitals in hotels at Helouan, a health and thermal spa town well known to British tourists, which was 26 kilometres south of Cairo, and another near the sea at Alexandria.[91] Egypt's magnificent tourist hotels were essentially taken over during the war years by the WO either as hospitals or as accommodation for army and medical staff.

Lucy was fascinated by Egypt. When the medical staff was off duty, they became tourists just like the encamped soldiers and she was entranced by the mixture of ancient culture and the frenetic activity of war. Lucy walked through streets smelling of camels and donkeys and crowded with soldiers, nurses, transport wagons and ambulances. She explored winding and intersecting lanes filled with shops selling curios; scarabs and figurines both genuine and fake, and postcards. Major George Bourne, for example, wrote to his sister Eleanor that he was sending home parcels of souvenirs that he felt were of 'real antiquity', and in Australian homes every-where, postcards were displayed on mantelpieces and then pasted into family photo albums. From Saladin's Citadel, Lucy could see dozens of mosques; their architecture, windows and alabaster she thought wondrous. Entering one of the mosques, she found Punjabi Sikhs of the British army inside, using the tiled cool space for their prayers.

During her time in Cairo there were often German planes overhead but Lucy felt that their bombing attempts would make no real impression on the 'flying sands' of the desert.[92] Both medical staff and the patients in Egypt had always to deal with the oppressive heat, which on some days in April, May and June could be excoriating. The wind, known as the Khamsin, delivered a fiery blast and sand blew into everything. Temperatures could reach 44.4°C on these days. With the evacuation of the Gallipoli Peninsula completed by late December 1915, the demand for medical care was beginning to decline in Egypt. By March 1916, both Lucy and Dr Agnes Bennett, who had been in Egypt serving in New Zealand and British hospitals for almost a year, began to consider moving on.

Eastern Front: Petrograd, Russia

November 1915, Autumn

Dr Laura Forster's work in Belgium came to an end in the spring of 1915 and later in the year she set out from London to reach Petrograd (St Petersburg) in Russia. It was a journey of more than 2000 kilometres but distance and difficulty never seemed to bother Laura. She set out independently, to work in Petrograd's terribly understaffed hospitals. A sea and train trip for the intrepid, it took at least nine days to reach Petrograd and regularly involved rough seas and dreadful seasickness. Laura would have travelled by train to either Newcastle, to join the SS *Bessheim*, a passenger and mail ship owned by the Norwegian Fred Olsen Line, or to Dundee in Scotland to sail on the SS *The Balder*, a Swedish Lloyd Company ship. Dundee was the British port closest to Norway but ships from all British ports en route to Petrograd travelled regularly through Bergen and Christianssand (Kristiansand) in Norway's south. These were small mail steamers with capacity for 110 passengers that sailed across the North Sea to the south coast of Norway and on to the Danish capital of Copenhagen, zigzagging to avoid detection by German U-boats. Then, coming perilously close to the northern coast of Germany, they steamed north into the Baltic Sea to Sweden's capital, Stockholm.

The direct route from Stockholm would have been due east to Petrograd but the German navy dominated the approach to the Russian city in order to prevent the Allies from supplying the Russians through the port. They had also laid mines in the Baltic to provide flanking cover from Allied shipping as the German army advanced north along the Baltic coast.[93] Instead of travelling east, passenger boats had to steam 1000 kilometres north into the Gulf of Bothnia, hugging the coast of Sweden, all the way to the port of Haparanda. There, Laura would have taken a Sami sleigh ride drawn by reindeer across the bridges to Tornea in Lapland (Tornio, now in Finland) and boarded a train to travel back in the opposite direction. After a trip of seven to nine days, her train would finally reach Petrograd, 1000 kilometres to the south, in Russia.[94] Sometimes even this route was too dangerous.

The only alternative was to take the lengthy trip up the west coast of Norway into the unpredictable seas and Arctic weather of the Norwegian Sea and the North Cape (Nordkapp). On 6 November 1915 a group of doctors and nurses heading to the Anglo–Russian Hospital in Petrograd took this route and it is possible that Laura was with them. The boats travelled

> between the Shetlands, Iceland, and the grim Norwegian coast deep cut with fjords and dented by the eternal succession of Atlantic gales . . . beneath the lace light of the Northern Lights.[95]

Storms and gales were common and almost everyone would be horribly seasick. Typically the boats stopped at Hönningsvåg in Norway and Murmansk in Russia before heading south into the White Sea to land at Archangel (Arkhangelsk). This was followed by a 1200-kilometre train trip before they finally arrived in Petrograd.[96] For the boat trip, Laura would have worn a waterproof cloak or leather coat padded and lined with sheepskin over her long coat and dress as well as fur-lined boots. The group likened their appearance to Tweedledum and Tweedledee in battle array![97] In early November, temperatures fell to below zero overnight, daylight lasted for just six hours and ice covered the rails and decks in the mornings. Between September and November, five German U-boats harassed Allied shipping and by Christmas, floating ice was preventing entry into Archangel's harbour. While Laura's boat made it through to Russia, further trips from England had to be postponed until the spring of 1916.

In 1915, Russia's hospitals were under intense pressure both as a result of military action and the vast humanitarian disaster unfolding as the winter set in. The dislocation of war had caused millions of people to flee since the first few weeks of combat in late 1914, and refugees from Galicia and eastern Poland swarmed into Russia, adding to the local population's war woes. Galicia was situated perilously between the Russian Empire to the east and the Austro–Hungarian Empire to the west and became the battleground for invasion by both sides.[98] In the second half of 1915 an estimated 3 million people headed into Russia, often with little food and few belongings.[99] In December 1915, the NUWSS responded to an appeal from the Tatiana Refugee Committee in Moscow by raising £5000 to fund a maternity hospital for refugee mothers, which opened in Petrograd in February 1915. Laura's love for both adventure and the chance to practise her surgical skills saw her arrive in the city late in 1915 and by December she was working in the men's surgical department of the city's largest hospital.

With a real talent for languages, in a short space of time Laura had readily learned enough Russian to work with the local doctors and patients without the need for interpreters.

London, England

Early 1916

Dr Elizabeth Hamilton-Browne thought she could put her skills in anatomy and physiology to good use for the war effort and late in 1915 decided to volunteer her services in London to the Society of Friends. Elizabeth graduated with first class honours at a University of Sydney Commemoration in April 1910, and anatomy was her forte. Elizabeth was a Quaker and the Quakers had set up The Friends' Ambulance Unit in the early months of the war. They considered that ambulance provision early in the war was distressingly inadequate and had established field ambulances and an ambulance train in 1915. Early in 1916 they added a Friends' hospital ship. This enabled Quakers to contribute without compromising their belief in non-violence. If the Friends could not accept her offer, Elizabeth thought she would volunteer at any Australian military hospital that would accept her services.

She sailed through the Heads of Sydney Harbour on 20 November 1915 on a general cargo ship, the SS *Sussex*, bound for London via Melbourne, Adelaide and Durban. The *Sussex* was a small boat and the trip took ten weeks, made a little longer by a slight collision with a coal ship in the Channel, off the eastern coast of Kent. By early 1916 the Channel shipping lanes were packed with troop, hospital, coal and cargo ships, all zigzagging to avoid German U-boats. Elizabeth paid her way by acting as the Ship's Doctor, for which she received a nominal 3d (three pence) at the end of the trip.[100]

Elizabeth wrote to her anatomy and physiology professor Sir Thomas Anderson Stuart from her room in Princes Square, close to Hyde Park and Kensington Palace, late in February 1916. His letter of introduction had helped her to meet Dr Flora Murray at the Endell Street Military Hospital and Elizabeth had been taken on as a surgeon with a nominal rank of lieutenant under the Chief Surgeon Dr Louisa Garrett Anderson. She was still finding her way around 'this enormous city' and had met up with Elsie Dalyell, who would have liked to return to work in Serbia had the situation there not been so catastrophic.[101] Elizabeth began work at the Endell Street Hospital in March 1916 and was joined a few weeks later by one of her Sydney University colleagues, Dr Eleanor Bourne.

Throughout 1915, women doctors had been rejected by the military when they attempted to enlist, but they had nevertheless been providing their expertise and experience to voluntary medical services. By the end of that year, there were ten Australian women doctors working overseas. They wrote home to their colleagues and inspired others to buy a ticket to London and war work.

Part 3

1916

Chapter 3

'The bullets were singing all over the field'[1]

It was wonderful to be hailed by our own boys from the bank
of the Suez Canal and they, in turn, were 'hailed' by us with
cigarettes, oranges, etc.[2]

Dr Eleanor Bourne, Egypt, April 1916

London, England

April 1916, Spring

Dr Eleanor Bourne had been thrilled to receive an appointment
to the surgical staff of the Endell Street Military Hospital early
in 1916 and sailed for England on HMAT *Malwa* on 21 March
1916. Eleanor had excelled in her secondary education, topping
the state of Queensland and scooping up several academic prizes
in 1896. An outstanding student at Brisbane Girls' Grammar,
she had to attend the Boys' Grammar in Forms 5 and 6 in order
to study Latin and Advanced Mathematics.[3] She was awarded a
government exhibition for entrance to the University of Sydney,
the first to be given to a woman. Eleanor graduated in medicine
in 1903.

Her decision to seek leave from her position as the first medical officer for Queensland's schools arose for several reasons. Firstly, she wanted to do her duty as a trained surgeon; she was excited by the prospect of working with leading women medical specialists at the Endell Street Military Hospital and she knew that her brother, Lieutenant Colonel George Bourne, was recuperating in London from illness contracted at Gallipoli.

Eleanor travelled in a saloon cabin, but below decks were around 300 soldiers, most of whom were reinforcements for the AIF's 23rd and 24th Infantry Battalions. By July and August 1916, they would be fighting in the bloody battles for Pozieres and Mouquet Farm in France. The ship also carried much-needed exports to England, including 800 cases of fruit and over 1000 boxes of soap. Sailing along the Suez Canal, Eleanor was delighted to see Australian soldiers camped along the banks. They came out to wave at the ship and the passengers threw oranges and packets of cigarettes to 'our own boys'.[4] Sighting seaplanes for the first time at Port Said, she wrote that they looked like graceful seabirds as they alighted around their warships.

The *Malwa* zigzagged through the Mediterranean and crept along the north coast of Crete during the day to avoid enemy ships, while a choppy sea with mist and rain apparently discouraged German submarines. On arriving in England on 28 April, they were greeted by a brief air-raid as German airships bombed England's southern coast and parts of London. Eleanor was shocked by newspaper reports of the Irish Easter rebellion, having taken the unity of Empire for granted. She had four days until her work began on 1 May at Endell Street.

When Eleanor arrived in May 1916, the Endell Street Hospital had at least 560 beds, with another 230 in attached auxiliary hospitals. There were more than 180 staff, all but six or seven being female.[5] The hospital stood in the middle of London and, being close to the city's main railway stations, received many seriously wounded soldiers brought from the ambulance trains arriving from France. Eleanor's daily surgical experiences included major abdominal surgery and many cases where the weaponry of World War I had caused devastating destruction to bones, frequently in the leg, and accompanying damage to surrounding tissues.

Amputation was a surgical procedure that Endell Street's surgeons had to quickly become accustomed to performing. Eleanor's Australian colleague Dr Vera Scantlebury said of her first few months at the hospital that she was finding military surgery 'truly awful'.[6] Despite the initial trauma of the work, Eleanor found it both a pleasure and an inspiration to be associated with 'so many splendid women'.[7] Dr Flora Murray, a tall, calm and unhurried woman, was the chief physician and took care of much of the administration, including the endless 'purple papers' of instructions from the WO and army paperwork. Dr Louisa Garrett Anderson, smaller and known for her quick movements and energy, was the chief surgeon. The hospital had a number of specialists, including a brilliant pathologist, Dr Helen Chambers, and an extremely busy radiologist, Dr Ethel Magill, who located a prodigious number of pieces of shrapnel with great skill, enabling the surgeons to achieve better results.

At first Eleanor lived in a flat just north of the British Museum, a fifteen-minute walk through Russell Square to the hospital. But after a while she found the long unending lines of terrace houses depressing and moved to a hotel behind Selfridge's large department store, which had been taken over by the WO's Department of Provisions. It was further away from the hospital but close to Hyde Park and Eleanor was keen to live in proximity to the green and relative quiet of London's parks. She was fascinated by the many characters that lived in the hotel, including Sir Patrick Manson, commonly known as the 'father of tropical medicine'. There was also a group of three, said to have fled from Russia, who owned a forbidding bulldog and a parrot. When the trio disappeared one night, 'Polly was left to foot the bill.'[8] It was here, from the roof of the hotel, that Eleanor watched a German Zeppelin airship fall burning from the sky and she was on duty when the hospital was showered with pieces of burnt paper from a hit on the nearby London General Post Office.

Kent, England

1915–1916, Winter
Dr Isabella Younger arrived in London from working in Glasgow and Edinburgh some time during 1915 to work at the 150-year-old Lying-In Hospital near Waterloo Station. Isabella came from the Victorian country town of Warrnambool on the state's south-west coastline but, after starting her medical degree in Melbourne, she had completed her final year of studies at the University of Glasgow in 1914.

Waterloo Station was one of the critical centres for arriving wounded and, when not at the maternity hospital, Isabella would visit the teeming station to offer assistance as the patients were unloaded from their ambulance trains and into waiting Red Cross ambulances.[9] Motor ambulances had never been used in war before 1914, and in the first weeks the wounded were transported in uncomfortable horse-drawn wagons or large motor trucks and were often painfully bumped and jostled along. *The Times* of London ran a fundraising campaign and in three weeks during October 1914 raised enough funds to buy 512 ambulances.

The British Red Cross also established a motor ambulance section and, over the course of the war, sent almost 2200 motor ambulances throughout the war zones.[10] Red Cross volunteers unloaded the trains and drove the ambulances and, as the war continued, more and more women became ambulance drivers. Few women had driven an automobile or a motorcycle before the war but critical need quickly overcame the old social mores.

Isabella approached Dr Louisa Garrett Anderson at Endell Street Military Hospital, offering to undertake surgical work. Having gained second class honours in physiology and anatomy in the final year of her medical degree, Isabella felt she could contribute, but Louisa suggested she help with the medical problems of the civilian population instead.[11] This was probably because Isabella was a new graduate and her most recent work experience was in children's and women's hospitals, which were also desperately short of medical staff.

In 1916, Isabella worked at a Kent military hospital, possibly the one established in the converted Royal Sailor's Rest. The county of Kent was closest to the Belgian and French coast and the hospital was the first in England to take Belgian wounded in October 1914. Later it took British wounded. Over the course of the war, more than 2.5 million casualties arrived back in England, mostly through the Kentish ports. Although there are no details of the nature of Isabella's work, the hospital's history includes stories of the injuries suffered by their soldier patients and how they felt about reaching hospital. A Canadian soldier who described his experience wrote:

> It did seem strange, that charge across the fields, dark and cold, with a blowing rain; all sorts of queer frightening noises, too. It seemed wonderful I wasn't hit; I remember thinking

how very wonderful it was. The bullets were singing all over
the field . . . Just as I reached the wood – smash went my arm!
Like a dry stick breaking . . . felt numbed, very queer – not
exactly pain, or else pain too bad to be felt . . . And the noise
going on, groanings, and cries . . . then wet darkness. Scarcely
a third of our fellows left . . . Shattered wrist and forearm; it's
all written on that little board top of my bed.[12]

Machine gun bullets fractured bones in the arms and legs of
soldiers, and wires, metal plates and screws were used to stabilise
and connect the breaks. Isabella's work would have involved the
post-operative supervision of the surgery and checking carefully
for any sign of infection.

London, England

May 1916, Spring
In the spring of 1916, Elizabeth Hamilton-Browne and Eleanor
Bourne were joined at Endell Street by Dr Rachel Champion,
a University of Melbourne graduate. Like many of her female
colleagues, Rachel's final-year university results were outstanding,
with first class honours in surgery and clinical surgery. She shared
the Fulton Prize for Obstetrics and Gynaecology and won a P&O
scholarship for further study in England on graduating in April
1914.

By 1916, the war had been grinding on for two years. The
slaughter continued unabated and the demand for medical
services was enormous. On the Western Front, the first Battle of
the Somme, from July to November 1916, resulted in appalling
losses, with British and Commonwealth casualties of 420,000.

As a result, London military hospitals were constantly receiving convoys of wounded soldiers.

Rachel left Melbourne for London on the RMS *Orontes* and although it was late November in 1915, the overnight temperature was an unseasonable 4.8°C and rain had turned to hail. The *Orontes* was not officially a troopship until later in 1916 but AIF reinforcements were onboard, including Private Archibald Darling Gould.

Archie's parents had signed his permission form and he enlisted with the 12th Light Horse Regiment in Claremont, Tasmania, in late August 1915. On his enlistment form he entered his age as eighteen years and four months but Archie was barely five months past his seventeenth birthday. The *Orontes*, with both Rachel and the reinforcements on board, sailed via Colombo and Port Said, and Rachel would then cross the Mediterranean to Toulon in France and on through the Strait of Gibraltar to London. Archie and his unit left the boat at Port Said for training at Serapeum, 93 kilometres to the south where the Australian Light Horse Brigade was guarding the Suez Canal. By the end of June he was in France and on 13 August 1916, barely eight and a half months after boarding the *Orontes*, he was killed in action during the Battle of the Somme. He was eighteen years and four months old. HMATS *Benalla* brought a small parcel of his belongings home to his family eight months later. He has no known grave.[13]

Like most people who went to war, Rachel Champion had multiple motivations. As a recent graduate, she wanted to do her duty by providing her medical skills in a military hospital. But she also was keen to be reunited with her fiancé, Major (Dr) Gordon Shaw, who had enlisted in 1914, two weeks after war was declared. He arrived at Gallipoli on 5 April 1915, joining the hospital ship *Gascon* a month later, and by late 1916 he had become an operating surgeon with the 1st Australian Casualty Clearing Station at Boulogne and at Harefield in England.[14] In London, Rachel shared a flat with two elderly women in Golders Green, with its convenient Tube station for travelling to the Endell Street Military Hospital.

Napsbury, England

March 1916, Spring

After almost six months at the No. 2 Anglo–Belgian Military Hospital in Calais, France, Dr Katie Ardill returned to England in March 1916 to a posting at the County of Middlesex War Hospital at Napsbury, about 40 kilometres north of London. For Katie, her new posting was a pleasant change from the wooden huts and duckboards of the Calais hospital. The hospital was previously the Napsbury Asylum for mental patients and was built on Napsbury Manor Farm, retaining the kitchen gardens, orchard, glasshouses and the thatched dairy. Napsbury had made full use of the manor's pre-existing tall trees when it was opened in 1905 and it had beautifully landscaped gardens and grounds. Katie would have alighted at Shenley village station, 3 kilometres away, where Belgian and French soldiers were regularly unloaded from hospital trains, and arrived at the hospital's main building, which looked a lot like a gabled country mansion.

Napsbury continued its psychiatric work with soldiers suffering from mental illness. Of the 1520 beds at the hospital, 350 were reserved for these patients. Australian Sergeant Archie Barwick recorded the effect on his men's minds of a relentless artillery bombardment during the Battle of Pozieres in late July 1916. Many Australian trenches collapsed and soldiers had to be dug out. He wrote:

> All day long the ground rocked & swayed backwards and forwards from the concussion . . . Men were driven stark staring mad, & more than one of them rushed out of the trench, over towards the Germans. Any amount of them could be seen crying and sobbing like children, their nerves completely gone.[15]

Many Australian soldiers were cared for at Napsbury and Private TC Haynes from South Australia, admitted in the autumn of 1916 with trench fever, was a typical case. Trench fever was one of the major causes of illness in soldiers during World War I, and was transmitted by body lice that thrived in the confines of the Western Front trenches. In 1916, Katie had neither drugs nor vaccines to provide a cure for these fevers, so disinfection and rest in a clean and warm environment were the only treatments she could prescribe.

Western Front: Lyon, France

May 1916, Spring

Her four months of service in Egypt complete, Dr Lucy Gullett arrived in London in April 1916 and within weeks was appointed to the Hôpital d'Ulster for French soldiers in Lyon.[16] The Ulster Volunteer Force Medical and Nursing Corps of Belfast offered their services firstly to the WO, who declined. The French accepted the offer and the Ulster Volunteers raised the money to fund a hospital and ambulance in Pau in the south-west of France. They then opened a second hospital on 31 May 1915, in Lyon. Lucy arrived at the 100-bed Lyon hospital sometime in May 1916, during the fourth month of one of the largest battles on the Western Front – the Battle of Verdun.

It is estimated that 56,000 French soldiers were killed and
almost 200,000 wounded at Verdun. The wounded poured into
the city of Lyon, requiring 57,000 beds to be set up there.[17]
Soldiers arrived from the train with cardboard labels attached
to their clothing. A red label denoted severe wounds, blue less
severe but still serious, and white for milder injuries. As far as
was possible, orderlies – many of whom were young Catholic
priests – packaged up the soldiers' clothes, boots, helmets and
personal belongings. The enormous number of wounded meant
stations overflowed with soldiers and stretchers, and hospital
trains had to wait in lines that were sometimes over 8 kilometres
long. It often took thirty-six exhausting hours, and sometimes
longer, for wounded soldiers to reach Lyon after being picked up
from a casualty clearing station (CCS).

Lucy admired the bandaging that had been done in the pres-
sured haste of the CCSs close to the frontlines. The CCSs were
located in positions hopefully just beyond the range of the enemy's
guns and preferably near to transport. Often under fire, stretcher-
bearers brought the wounded to regimental aid posts where the
most urgently needed first aid was applied, especially for haemorrhage and pain control. The wounded men were then carried
to or placed in an ambulance to be moved on to the nearest CCS.
A team of surgeons and nurses would there stabilise the wounded
soldier so that he could be sent on to a field or military hospital like
the Hôpital d'Ulster in Lyon. Bathing, rebandaging and further
surgery, such as secondary amputation, could then take place but
it was the skill of the initial work that Lucy found amazing.

Different hospitals in Lyon specialised in a particular kind of
wound: facial, back, nervous and head. While the introduction of
helmets after the first few months of war reduced the death toll
from head injuries, Lucy said she treated injuries that resulted

when helmets were bent and twisted, and looked like sardine cans opened with a fork.[18]

Lucy returned home in late 1916 and continued to speak of the terrible damage done by shrapnel and how the broken, jagged pieces of metal tore into the soldiers' flesh, carrying pieces of mud-stained clothing with it and the possibility of tetanus and gas gangrene. She also said that wounded men who had lain for long periods in no-man's land surrounded by the roar of bursting shells were easily recognised in the hospital. They carried the signs of strain for many months.[19]

Cairo, Egypt

April 1916, Spring
Almost a year after Dr Agnes Bennett's arrival in Cairo, the pressing need for medical staff in Egypt eased and she decided it was time to move on to London, hoping to visit Helen Sexton in Paris on the way. But before leaving she got a pass to visit her brother Bob in Alexandria:

> It is just 7.45 a.m. and I am on my way to meet dear old Roberto . . . And it's just the most glorious day possible, a lovely fresh morning air coming in and all the villages alive with blue-gowned fellaheen marketing; dear little donks and groaning old camels.[20]

After her visit she wrote: 'One can't help feeling a bit sad, but there's gladness in it too, for the boy is looking just splendid.'[21]

Chapter 4

'At the bottom of a deep narrow shell wound'

So many of the cases . . . proved to have early gas formation
at the bottom of a deep narrow shell wound that it would
certainly be fatal to leave them; they would probably have lost
a limb, if not life.[1]

Dr Elsie Dalyell, France, July 1916

London, England

May 1916, Spring

Dr Agnes Bennett departed the Choubra Infectious Diseases
Hospital in Cairo in April 1916, arriving in London in early May.
Having tea at the Lyceum Club in Piccadilly she was delighted
to come across her friend Dr Elsie Inglis, who had been the dean
of her alma mater, the College of Medicine for Women at the
University of Edinburgh, during her studies. Elsie had recently
returned from the SWH units on the Eastern Front and the women
discussed the dire medical situation of the Serbian army and their
epic journey through the mountains in freezing conditions. The
Serbs had been unable to withstand Austria's second invasion of

their country in October 1915. But by the time Agnes arrived in London, the army had regrouped. With Allied help the Serbs were preparing to liberate their homeland, amassing their troops in Salonica to travel north through Greece and Macedonia.[2]

Elsie Inglis' Serbian SWH units were recuperating back in England after their enforced departure from the country, either as prisoners of war or as members of the appalling retreat through the mountains of Montenegro and Albania. Undaunted, Elsie was planning to dispatch another mobile field hospital to Serbia to support the revitalised Serbian army and she was looking for staff. Agnes was in total agreement with Elsie's continuing ambition to demonstrate the worth of women's work, later writing: 'This work is doing just what I have always so much wished to do – proving that women can organise and run such institutions from top to toe.'[3]

In May 1916 Agnes Bennett was appointed as CMO of the new SWH unit heading to Greece and given the task of establishing a base hospital in Salonica for the Third Serbian Army. It was to be called the America Unit, named for the country that had supplied the majority of the funds.[4]

Western Front: Royaumont, France

May 1916, Spring

Dr Elsie Dalyell also signed up with the SWH in 1916 following her eight months' work in the Addington Park Military Hospital's diagnostic laboratory at Croydon. In May Elsie travelled across the Channel to France, arriving by train at the SWH's Royaumont hospital just north of Paris, and within earshot of the guns on the Western Front that thundered day and night.[5]

The hospital had been recently created in the grand medieval Cistercian Abbey of Royaumont, built between 1229 and 1235 in the countryside near the villages of Asnières-sur-Oise and Viarmes. The abbey was privately owned by industrialist Edouard Goüin, who offered it for treatment of the wounded. The CMO and Chief Surgeon was 44-year-old Scot Dr Frances Ivens, a graduate of the LSMW. Like Elsie, she was an exceptional student and had graduated with first class honours.[6] Although the hospital was approved by the British and French Red Cross, the French military's initial response was very guarded and it was not until Royaumont's unflagging performance during the Battle of the Somme in mid-1916, that the French government embraced the hospital and its female staff.

Despite its outward attractiveness, vaulted corridors and cloisters, the abbey had no heating, furniture or electricity and only a trickle of water when the SWH women first arrived in the biting cold of December 1914. The massive stove had not been lit for ten years and they had to scrub the accumulated dirt from the floors and walls. Often they scrubbed by candlelight, moving the candles in their blue enamel holders as they toiled.[7] By the time Elsie arrived in 1916, many of the early building and supply challenges had been overcome, although the plumbing remained annoyingly unreliable.

Two aspects of the medical work at Royaumont piqued Elsie's interest. Firstly, the laboratory had been established by Scot Dr Elizabeth Butler who, like Elsie, had been awarded the prestigious Beit Fellowship. Elizabeth and Elsie were the two most eminent women scientists of the Empire pre-war. Secondly, Professor Weinberg of the Pasteur Institute in Paris, the leading expert on gas gangrene, had chosen Royaumont's lab from dozens of other military hospitals available to him to test his new gas gangrene anti-sera.

Also, Dr Ivens was aware of the work of Belgian surgeon Dr Antoine DePage, who believed that more soldiers' limbs and lives could be saved with improved wound management. She implemented his process where wounded patients had their wounds surgically cleaned (debrided) and dressed but not stitched until the results of swabs taken from the wounds by a pathologist such as Elsie were examined to identify anaerobic bacteria that could cause the frequently fatal gas gangrene. Surgical closure of the wounds did not take place until the bacteria had disappeared from the swabs. This was intensive and time-consuming. Australian nurse Leila Smith described this procedure when she worked in one of Wimereux's many military hospitals:

> I had a ward of 34 beds; every man had his bacterial chart as well as his temperature chart. The pathologist did the films and sent back a report on which we marked the chart up. When we got three negatives the wound was stitched up. The results were splendid. We had a great staff . . . charting etc took a lot of time.[8]

The work of all the medical staff at Royaumont with gas gangrene was a significant contribution to the treatment of the wounded from the battlefield and from May to October 1916, Elsie Dalyell was in charge of the bacteriological laboratory.[9]

Although these methods increased the chance of survival, Elsie's work was not always successful. In March 1917, the *British Medical Journal* published her paper on a 1916 case of gas gangrene.[10] A 23-year-old French soldier had been wounded in the left thigh by a shell fragment at Maurecourt on 14 September 1916. Although only 40 kilometres away, he did not reach Royaumont until three days later on 17 September and an operation at 7 pm found gangrenous skin and muscles between his entry and exit wounds. Following the DePage method, the gangrenous areas were excised and the wound left open but his condition worsened and on Thursday morning his leg was amputated above the wound. Sadly, the young man died five hours later. In her paper, Elsie discussed her attempts to discover why the young soldier had died. She continued to experiment on guinea pigs in the laboratory with the hope of improving later treatments. The war thus provided women doctors with their first opportunity to publish research papers on a range of surgical and treatment techniques in areas to which they had previously had very little access. The publication of academic papers was important because it provided evidence to a wide audience within the profession of the quality of the work of women doctors, and hopefully was another step toward professional acceptance.

By late June, the Royaumont women could hear the preliminary Allied bombardment of the German lines. This heralded the Battle of the Somme and Dr Ivens had been warned to expect a rush. When it came on 2 July, Royaumont's radiologist recorded: 'We have had a ghastly time of horrors since Sunday. Men badly wounded pouring in at the rate of 70 to 100 per day.'[11] In the first day, 127 badly wounded men arrived from the station at Creil 20 kilometres away, their condition so desperate that they could not be moved any further.[12] A second operating theatre was hastily set up in a ward kitchen and both theatres worked continuously for the first three days, with the staff snatching short periods of sleep when they could. For the first eight days of the battle, surgeons and doctors managed only two hours of sleep per night and the unreliable power supply meant they sometimes operated by candlelight.[13]

In her remote lab in the abbey's garrets, accessed by a spiral staircase, Elsie conducted 180 bacteriological examinations during that time and identified 112 cases of gas gangrene. She also lent a

hand in theatre whenever she could. The French medical authorities asked Dr Ivens to double the number of beds at Royaumont
immediately and, as it was summer, they were able to place 50 beds
in the abbey's cloisters and nearly 100 in the refectory, which had
been the staff dining room. Staff meals had to be eaten outside
and by November everyone wore their warmest coats to dinner,
with the cloisters lit by moonlight on cloudless nights. If they
were unable to reach the cloisters quickly at mealtimes, their food
became very cold. The abbey's enormous garrets were also used
for storing the patients' uniforms and possessions.

Military hospitals like Royaumont had to manage not only the
physical needs of their patients but also their clothing, possessions
and the medical and personal records required by the military
outlined in the WO's purple papers. On admission, soldiers
were given hot soup and cigarettes and although they sometimes
arrived with nothing at all, any baggage they had was labelled by
orderlies. Men not requiring immediate surgery were bathed and
given a bed, their uniforms and underclothes placed in numbered
sacks. In the early months the sacks were carried up five floors
to the garrets but later a block and pulley system was installed to
save the orderlies' backs.

Clothing was sorted, labelled and sent to the laundry, and the
men's treasures such as pipes, tobacco, letters, photos and war
'trophies' were carefully wrapped and returned to their owners.
Local women washed and mended the linen and Royaumont
staff repaired the uniforms with anything they had on hand.
An orderly (and writer) at Royaumont, Vera Collum, recorded
the pleasure on the men's faces when they saw their kit washed,
mended and folded and ready for them when they recovered.[14]
The administration of this system began with a small lined
one-penny notebook but soon developed into a systematic card

index to handle the records of the 8752 soldiers who passed through the hospital between 1915 and 1919.

A local factory owner, Monsieur Delacoste, heard that the women were eating their meals outside in the cold. He sent his men to build a wooden hut next to the abbey's main building and fitted it with a stove so that, by late November, the staff could eat inside and both staff and their food stayed warm. He also installed a new incinerator to cope with the enormous quantity of dressings – and the amputated limbs – that had to be disposed of.

This was the time before antibiotics, and thousands of amputations took place in World War I to save terribly wounded men from developing gas gangrene. The simplest form of amputation was a circular procedure with the wound left wide open. The first step was to tie off the artery and vein in the limb to prevent haemorrhage. The nerves were usually then pulled down, cut very short and crushed and tied. The muscles were then cut through, and finally the bone was manually sawn through using various-sized serrated implements depending on the site of the cut. More than 41,000 British soldiers had one or more limbs amputated during the war, causing them tremendous personal trauma. The procedure was challenging for doctors too. The emotional and physical debilitation for the women surgeons was only offset by the knowledge that they had often saved a man's life by amputating. Elsie's irrepressible optimism and renowned chuckle helped when the doctors were feeling disheartened and her 'quick-change impersonations of Scottish women in the incredible variety of tartan-trimmed garments which Edinburgh considered suitable as uniform were much appreciated'.[15]

Elsie was keen to broaden her pathology experience and laboratory research, and having served for six months at Royaumont, she departed to take up a position on the island of Malta.

Western Front: Limoges, France

June 1916, Summer

As the women at Royaumont were preparing for the rush from the Battle of the Somme, Dr Isabel Ormiston was once again put to work by the WARC. She had recuperated from the taxing journey on horseback through the Dinaric Alps to Salonica with a stay in the warmth of Alexandria in Egypt. For a short time she worked at one of the British Convalescent Depots there. At least seven or eight depots were established at Alexandria, Abbassia and Helouan (Helwan) in tents by the sea, in large grand hotels and in the Sultan's El Walda Palace which, much to the surprise of the patients, had its own zoo. Isabel returned to London for reassignment with the WARC.

During the first weeks of the war in late 1914, the WARC had cared for the Belgian wounded by requesting two ships for the transport of Belgian soldiers to England. However, by 1915 it was clear that the demand for medical services was huge and volunteers like the WARC had a much larger role to play in caring for wounded and sick soldiers and civilians close to the European battlefields. Although mostly WO approved, organisations like the WARC received little government assistance and they had to work throughout the war to raise the funds to keep their units and hospitals in the field. Fundraising was a massive enterprise with campaigns throughout the Empire and also in America.

By mid-1916 the WARC was running two hospitals in France: one was in Dieppe and the second was a 225-bed hospital in Limoges in the Musée Nationale de Céramique.[16] General Delorme, France's leading military surgeon and inspector of military hospitals, was impressed by the WARC's Limoges hospital, which received the wounded directly from the frontline, trans-ported in hospital trains.

The time taken for a wounded man to reach a military hospital from the battlefield could vary from several hours to several days but relief was sometimes provided by the Red Cross canteens set up by their volunteers along the major rail lines. They provided sweets, cigarettes, hot coffee, chocolate, soup and sometimes meals or hot snacks. The soldiers were especially glad to see them when they were lying on station platforms for hours at a time. Frequently, long and even overnight delays were caused by large convoys of wounded going in one direction and equally large numbers of rail trucks filled with soldiers, equipment and supplies going the other way.

Isabel was appointed to the Limoges WARC hospital, the Hôpital Militaire Anglais de Limoges, arriving in mid-1916. The hospital opened in October 1914 with accommodation for 150 to 160 patients. Being on the main railway line from Paris to Bordeaux, the hospital received their wounded from the frontline's casualty clearing stations within thirty to forty hours. The building was four storeys high and there was a great deal of climbing up and down stairs, carrying patients, supplies and meals. In 1917 the number of beds had increased to 305 and by December 1919 more than 11,000 sick and wounded soldiers had been treated there.

Norfolk, England

June 1916, Summer
As a young woman, Victorian Dr Irene Eaton decided to follow in her father's footsteps and study medicine. She completed her medical and surgical degrees at the LSMW in 1909, the year that

Grace Cordingley arrived from Sydney to enrol for her studies at the school. Irene's war service began sometime in 1916 at the Norfolk War Hospital in Norwich as an assistant pathologist, where she ran the tests concerned with assessing a soldier's fitness for returning to France. RAMC medical boards had to decide whether a soldier's rehabilitation should be continued or whether he was fit for active service, fit only for light duties or had a permanent disability caused by his war service. In the last case his pension entitlements had to be determined.

Returning men to the front was not an easy decision to make. Dr Flora Murray from the Endell Street Hospital was disturbed by:

The pathos of slight cases who had to be sent back and that the soldiers were given a parcel and a good send-off but there was no getting over the horror of going back.[17]

In the first week of August 1916, Irene joined the first group of women doctors to leave for Malta to work for the RAMC in the island's hospitals; she was one of twenty-one on board.

Malta

August 1916, Summer
Until the spring of 1916, the British WO had been affronted by any change in perceived pre-war gender roles and concerned to prevent women other than nurses from entering the military sphere. As Dr Flora Murray, co-founder of the Endell Street Military Hospital, put it: 'In August 1914 it was a popular idea that war was man's business and that everything and everyone should stand aside and let men act.'[18]

However, the war's voracious demand for personnel of every kind on both the home and battle fronts, and the unrelenting consumption of medical resources, led to a re-examination of women's wartime roles. In May 1916, Lieutenant General Keogh, Director General of Medical Services, made a significant request of the Dean of the LSMW, Dr Louisa Aldrich-Blake. Could she write to women doctors to encourage them to work for the RAMC in Malta, Egypt and in British hospitals?

Louisa wrote to all of the women on the British Medical Register and initially forty-eight came forward to enrol. There was no question of the women enlisting, their rank being gazetted or them being given an RAMC uniform with insignia of rank. Indeed, it was not until April 1918 that women doctors were permitted to wear a uniform with an RAMC badge pinned to each lapel.[19] Driven by necessity, the WO was prepared to hire women doctors but would not allow them access to 'the complex codes of rank, decorations and uniforms that are awarded . . . after various rites of passage'.[20] Without rank, their place in a military hospital hierarchy was dependent on the particular attitude of each CO to women doctors.

Women doctors were to be classified as 'civilian surgeons' attached to the RAMC and given a twelve-month contract at 24 shillings per day. A £60 gratuity was paid at the contract's end as long as the doctor had not been dismissed for misconduct.[21] By the end of the war, the RAMC would have employed women doctors to work all over Britain and in Egypt, but the early groups were sent to the rocky, sunny little island of Malta, a long way from any frontline.

Despite its distance from the frontline, Malta's hospitals treated more than 138,000 soldiers over the course of the war. The hospitals in Malta, along with those in Egypt, took the casualties from the Gallipoli campaign for nine months from April 1915 to January 1916. Hospital ships like HMHS *Gascon*, formerly a Union-Castle passenger liner, evacuated the wounded and hundreds of soldiers sick with dysentery and malaria from Gallipoli. The trip to Malta took five to six days. From October 1915, Malta's hospitals also took the wounded and sick from the Eastern Front battles via the port of Salonica, and continued to do so for almost three years.

Over three years, eighty-five women doctors served on Malta, including Australian doctors Irene Eaton, who set sail with the first group on 2 August 1916; Eveline Cohen a few weeks later in September; and Elsie Dalyell after she had completed her time with the SWH at Royaumont Abbey in early October 1916.

The hospital ships that brought the women doctors to Malta from England transited through Salonica and Mudros (Moudros), the port on the Greek island of Lemnos and the closest Allied hospital facility to the Gallipoli Peninsula. The ships landed soldiers returning to their units and picked up soldier patients at ports along the way. They also stopped several times to take on coal. Arriving at the Grand Port of Valetta on Malta, the women saw a breathtaking panorama of forts and great square, flat-roofed buildings atop massive stone walls that disappeared down into the sea. Washing hung from the front balconies of the apartment blocks that ran along Valetta's winding streets. At the dockside, a long row of Red Cross ambulances waited for the sick and wounded to be unloaded from the myriad ships and boats that crowded the harbour.[22] When Elsie Dalyell arrived later in 1916, her hospital accommodation was not ready and she was able to enjoy the sights of Valetta whilst staying in a small *pensione*.

They worked mostly at the 1158-bed St Andrews Hospital, a building of imposing architecture that overlooked St George's

Bay, and also at St David's, St George's and Valetta Hospitals. There were another twenty hospitals and convalescent camps on the island. VAD and writer Vera Brittain wrote of her hospital:

> Tuesday 24 October [St George's Hospital, Malta]
> This is a most beautiful hospital, built on a peninsula of land running right out into the sea . . . The sea is right below the rocks but there is a delightful little bay which is quite safe and very shallow though full of large fish; here we have our bathing place, and it is so near that we can go down from our rooms with mackintoshes over our bathing dresses.[23]

The larger hospitals were converted stone buildings but all were supplemented with concrete-floored marquees capable of holding ten to twenty beds each. Irene, Eveline and Elsie's work on the island was mainly with soldiers who were ill rather than wounded. The sick greatly outnumbered the wounded, with malaria, dysentery and different enteric fevers predominating. The only treatment for malaria was a regimen of quinine but it had to be administered consistently and could have side-effects, some of which were very dangerous. The island's OC noted that '42 medical women had arrived in Malta for duty, a most welcome reinforcement and an innovation attended in every way with the happiest results'.[24]

Eastern Front: Ostrovo, Macedonia

September 1916, Autumn
Back in Scotland, Dr Agnes Bennett had spent weeks interviewing nurses, orderlies and drivers, organising supplies and a fleet of

model-T Ford vehicles, which used up a lot of the American-raised funds. Heading up the SWH's America Unit, she sailed for Salonica on 3 August 1916 with the fifty-five female members of her field hospital, including one Scottish and three English women doctors, and Dr Jessie Scott, a colleague from New Zealand. They arrived safely ten days later.

Her unit was accompanied by members of the SWH's transport column, which was headed by Mrs Katherine Harley, a woman of forceful personality who was said to be a law unto herself. Agnes worried about the women with the Harley unit and thought their behaviour very unruly. She disapproved of them smoking in public, especially cigars, and her tolerance was greatly tested on the ship.

While internal discipline varied between units, Agnes took the issue of discipline very seriously and was keenly aware of her leadership role and her responsibility for the health and welfare of the women in her charge. She was also keenly aware that the behaviour of women in uniform was under constant scrutiny by both the public and the military, and within three months, the women of the transport unit were placed under Agnes' authority.

In Salonica, Agnes discovered that the plans for her unit had changed. The fighting was now in Macedonia and a hospital was needed closer to the action – in the hills at Lake Ostrovo (Lake Vegoritida, Greece), 140 kilometres north-west of Salonica.[25] There were delays in receiving the equipment and stores and, while waiting for almost three weeks, Agnes set up a temporary canteen for the soldiers at the Salonica railway station.

On 7 September the America Unit and its transport column set off from Salonica over the rugged mountains for Lake Ostrovo. They were planning to be within reach when the Serbian army tried to regain their homeland by fighting their way to Mount Kajmakčalan (Mt Kaimaktsalan, Greece). The doctors accompanying Agnes Bennett included Dr Jessie Scott and several British women doctors.

As they approached Ostrovo, Agnes thought their position was picturesque, with snow on the mountains all around them and the lake to one side. But later she wrote that the roads were so bad that fourteen of the staff had gone out one day with picks, shovels and barrows, to try to make it passable for the hospital's cars.[26] Finally arriving at Ostrovo after at least eight hours of travel over mountainous terrain with the unit's convoy of vehicles, staff and equipment, Agnes discovered that most of their advance party had succumbed to malaria and were of little help.

Her group's first task was to create a workable camp and hospital under the available trees. Before the unit's arrival, a horse-drawn artillery unit had been camped there and the whole site had to be cleared. They could then set about erecting their large, heavy, wooden-floored tents, and Agnes directed the digging of drainage channels and the first sewage pits.

Once the tents were up, the stores of medical equipment, utensils, beds, blankets and food could be unpacked. Over eleven days the camp gradually took shape, although Agnes was anxious that the disinfector had not yet arrived.[27] Once the camp was established, she wrote of her unbounded admiration for the committee back in Edinburgh. The equipment they provided – from petrol generators for electric light and radiography, right down to safety pins for bandages – showed tremendous planning and experience and Agnes received congratulations from visitors for their entire hospital installation.[28]

On 12 September 1916 the battle for the Gorničevo ridge began in the foothills of the Voras Mountains, in an area about 25 kilometres from Ostrovo – the first step on the way to Kajmakčalan, the mountain pass back into Serbia. The day before, the road in front of the hospital had been a caravanserai of pack mules and mounted Serbian soldiers. The day after, the parade included British supply lorries, carts driven by Serbs and French cavalry and 'Serbs providently leading sheep or goats with them, one with a lamb over his shoulders, and one with a black bantam on a string'.[29]

From the door of her tent, Agnes watched as shells curved through the sky heralding the start of a two-day artillery barrage against the Bulgarian enemy. The Third Serbian Army, camped not far from Ostrovo, fought their way up to the Gorničevo ridge, which gave access into the mountains. The unit's first patients were admitted five days later.[30]

We took about 24 cases, all terribly bad wounds, abdominal, chest, head, and compound fractures. It was terrible to see the poor fellows up at the dressing station. Five died before or just on arrival at the hospital. It was really a terrible day.[31]

As the Serbian army pushed forward, the trip to pick up the wounded became longer and longer, taking four to five hours and more when driving at night. Women ambulance drivers of the transport column drove their heavy Ford ambulances along narrow mule tracks that were now pitted with shell holes and tried to keep the awful lurching to a minimum for their patients. Other wounded were brought to the hospital by very primitive means. Sometimes they were transported in large conical baskets carried on either side of donkeys and sometimes on springless carts over the terribly rough roads. Sometimes the wounded were enemy soldiers.

Wed. Sept. 20th ... The poor Bulgar is terribly cut up. Compound fracture of thigh and mutilated right hand which had to be amputated. I took a big bit of shrapnel out of the thigh and quantities of wad. I think I may be able to save it but the hand had to go.[32]

Much to Agnes' relief, Dr Lilian Cooper from Brisbane arrived within a few days to bolster the medical team. With her was her companion, Miss Josephine Bedford, an ambulance driver who also had very handy mechanical skills. Lilian was an unusually tall woman who decided at the age of fifty-five to join the SWH and go to the war.[33] British by birth, but an Australian resident for twenty-five years, she was well used to travel and, as Australia's first fully qualified female surgeon, she was also well fitted for war surgery. Lilian was an exceptionally strong-minded woman. She studied medicine at the LSMW, the only medical school that accepted women students in England in the 1880s, beginning in 1886 and graduating in 1890. Although the school was part of the University of London, the university would not allow women to be admitted to degrees. With this in mind, and simultaneously with her London studies, she successfully completed the conjoint examinations for the Royal Colleges of Physicians and Surgeons in both Edinburgh and Glasgow and was admitted to both degrees.[34] Following advice from Dr Elizabeth Garrett Anderson, England's first registered woman doctor, Lilian travelled to Australia to take up a position as an assistant in a Brisbane practice. Unfortunately, this was a disastrous appointment and Lilian successfully sued for a release of her contract. As a result, she was professionally boycotted for the following two years. However, with her medical skills and determination she was able to set up her own practice in late 1891 and in 1896 was the first woman doctor in Australia to be appointed as a hospital honorary at the Brisbane Hospital for Sick Children.[35]

The battles for the ridge raged until the end of September and casualties poured into the unit's hospital.[36] Many men were dying on the hillsides as they waited to be picked up by ambulances that could not reach them in such inaccessible territory. For weeks there was not an empty bed in the hospital.[37] By 25 September the hospital had 160 cases and Agnes reported to the SWH headquarters in Edinburgh that the wounds were of the worst possible variety and often multiple. Gangrene was rife and the constant amputations were a terrible trial in the operating tent for both patient and surgeon.[38] On the last day in September 1916, every bed and blanket was taxed to the utmost.

The Serbian army required that Agnes' hospital be consecrated, or in other words receive a blessing, and in October, the Serbian Crown Prince Alexander and the Director of Serbian Medical Services, Colonel Sondermeyer, attended the consecration by a local priest attired in a gorgeous heavily embroidered gold robe. Although Agnes was a little put out at this interruption to the hospital's work, in the end she thought it was 'a great day' and the patients were honoured to meet the prince as he toured the wards.[39] The hospital now had 200 beds with ten patients in each tent ward, a reception tent for triage, as well as X-ray and dispensary tents. Agnes liaised constantly with Colonel Sondermeyer, attempting to stay informed about the battles and likely wounded.

The hospital treated soldiers from the Allied armies – Serbs, French, Canadians, Russians, Americans, Greeks, Moroccans, Italians and British – as well as some injured enemy soldiers – Germans, Austrians and Bulgarians. It was a camp of around fifty women, aged between twenty-five and fifty-five years, next to the railway line and surrounded by army camps. The frontline was 20 to 25 kilometres away and the roar of the guns led Agnes to write in January 1917 that 'the bombardment is continuous and sometimes seems to be so close that I feel very anxious'.[40] Everyone was shocked when they heard of the death of Katherine Harley two months later. Having been relieved of her duties with the transport column, Katherine had set up a small orphanage at Monastir (now Bitola, Macedonia), about 45 kilometres to the east of Agnes' hospital. She was killed in the town by shrapnel from an enemy bombardment on 8 March 1917.

At Ostrovo the doctors performed surgery, while other staff nursed, drove ambulances, maintained the motor vehicles and sanitary arrangements and worked as cooks and orderlies. They also had the assistance of some elderly Serbian men as orderlies. The ambulance drivers saw both the worst and the best of Serbia. They loaded the badly wounded into the ambulances and drove over rugged mountains only to find at times that their passengers had died. Finding enough petrol was a constant worry, the cars continually needed repairs for broken axles, hubs and transmissions, and spare parts were exceedingly difficult to obtain. But they also had the freedom of the open road, the spectacular scenery and occasionaly trips to the bustling and exotic city of Salonica.

With her usual optimism, Agnes, whom everyone called 'The Chief', wrote that the nurses 'really are splendid, never flinch at anything, and the staff are really working like bricks'.[41] In the first eight weeks the hospital admitted 523 cases with sixty deaths occurring.[42] There were also staff losses – in early October 1916, the staff mourned the loss of masseuse Olive Smith, who died from malaria; and later in 1917, one of the nurses, Sister Caton, died. On both occasions, the camp came to a standstill as the funerals were held. The burial of their colleagues took a heavy emotional toll.[43] Typhus also seriously tested everyone's physical and emotional resilience. Staff and patients battled flies, wasps and malaria-carrying mosquitoes in summer. Agnes wrote:

> Life in the Balkans is full of incident. On top of all our other troubles we had to contend with no end of pests, one of the worst of which were the wild dogs, like wolves, that used to keep up a monotonous baying all night and stealing our food unless we hung it out of their reach. Field mice used to eat our kit bags and our clothes: there were wasps in thousands: there were earwigs in millions.[44]

Nurses and doctors endured severe frosts and heavy snow in winter and performed surgery, often complex, in all weather and at all times of the day and night.

> Thursday, 16, XI, 16
>
> The weather is really miserable, snow on all the mountains round about, a cutting wind, and rain and mud underfoot . . . The Serbs know pretty well how to keep the cold out. One good dodge of theirs was to cut a petrol tin in half (4 gallon one) in two [sic] and fill one half with glowing ashes from the fire and stand it on top of the other . . . I have one almost under my nose.[45]

While the workload was often relentless, mundane and routine, there were also many brighter times for all of the staff at Ostrovo. Agnes and Lilian had an enjoyable social life with visits from Serbs, Frenchmen, Russians and Italians. Sometimes there were Greek soldiers and Macedonian civilians (who might be Romanian or Turkish) and a few black French colonels.[46] When they had spare time, the doctors rode horses and the staff explored the beautiful countryside and villages on foot, and Christmas was special, with a hilarious dress-up party and festive lunch. There were regular music concerts and visits from neighbouring soldiers' camps and Serbian dignitaries.

Agnes knew from her hospital's first days that delays caused by transporting wounded men for 22 kilometres over rough tracks from the frontline to the hospital increased both the death rate and the patients' terrible suffering. Just before Christmas 1916, she obtained permission from the local Serbian commander to set up a dressing station in the mountains at Dobraveni, much closer to the battle.[47]

Agnes and her staff were keen to relieve the soldiers' suffering and gave little consideration to their own safety. One of the orderlies wrote of the trips up to the Dobraveni dressing station, that they were an awful climb with rough and narrow tracks and the car engines constantly boiling. The view back over the Macedonian plains and Lake Ostrovo was wonderful and there were 'throngs of transport of many nations – Serbs, French, British, native Turks and Macedonians. Donkeys, mules, oxen, horses, carts, Ford vans and our ambulances.'[48] Whenever they stopped, children in the villages would lift the hems of the skirts worn by the drivers and orderlies to see what they had on their legs. And they wanted to know if the women had hair under their caps.

Conditions at Dobraveni were primitive and by the start of winter the weather was freezing. A small tent hospital with thirty-nine beds was set up in very rough terrain on the side of the mountain. Being close to the frontline, it was surrounded by dugouts, or 'funk holes', for protection from bombing raids. They built a kitchen from local stones with a chimney fashioned from kerosene tins and old petrol tins filled with soil; the roof was a tarpaulin.[49] Wounded men were brought in to the dressing station, treated and then transported by the unit's ambulances down the mountain to the Ostrovo hospital. Due to the intensity of the work and the severity of the conditions, staff members were rotated every six weeks.

> At times the roar of cannon is audible and the flash of the guns and star shells are visible after dark, and during the day the anti-aircraft guns are frequently busy driving off enemy aeroplanes. These hitherto have rigorously respected the large red cross on a background of many white sheets pegged in the ground in the middle of the camp.[50]

Winter snow and bitter winds, which sometimes reached gale force, were a major challenge at Dobraveni and keeping warm was a daily struggle. The cold hampered surgery as the operating fluids had to be thawed out before the surgeons could make a start, and they abandoned hospital whites, instead wearing as many layers of clothing as they could possibly work in. Heavy rains turned the surrounding ground into a mud pile and keeping everything clean and dry was a challenge.

Very thin and patrician in appearance, Dr Lilian Cooper was nevertheless well liked, and known not just for her surgical skills but for her propensity for using bad language under stress. This was something Agnes found difficult, but she very much appreciated Lilian's and Josephine's work. Lilian was also very popular with the young women drivers of the transport unit, who revelled in the freedom she encouraged; many had taken up smoking, and they insisted on wearing trousers and cutting their hair very short.

The women's happiness at their freedom contrasted and alleviated the seriousness and tragedies of their work. They loaded desperately wounded patients into the ambulances, and drove them along ravines on rocky tracks, often having to get out and push the vehicles when they became bogged in deep potholes. They had to repair the vehicles so often that Josephine became known as 'Miss Spare Parts'.[51] Under emergency conditions they worked very efficiently and effectively, tirelessly backing up Lilian's surgical work. Working in the pre-antibiotics era, Lilian found bomb wounds to be the worst as so many patients developed gas gangrene and it was very difficult to do anything with their wounds.

Epsom, England

August–November 1916, Autumn
During the four years of war, medical staff dealt with death almost daily but many also had to cope with overwhelming personal loss. Australian doctor Mary De Garis came to work with the SWH as a result of the loss of her fiancé, Sergeant Colin Thomson, in France in the summer of 1916. Having had her application for enlistment refused by the Australian army in 1915, Mary had decided in mid-1916 to put an end to her anxiety about Colin, and sailed to London to work at the Manor War Hospital.

Mary had completed her medical degree at the University of Melbourne in 1905 and was the second Victorian woman to obtain her Doctorate in Medicine in 1907. She worked twice in distant, isolated outback towns, firstly at Muttaburra in central Queensland in 1906–1907 and then in the far north-western corner of New South Wales at Tibooburra in 1911–1914. In Tibooburra she met and became engaged to Colin just as the war began.

Colin had survived Gallipoli but in mid-1916 he was deployed on the Western Front in France. Mary arrived in London on 14 July 1916 but soon after, Colin's postcards from the frontline stopped arriving. Her worst fears were realised when, in late September, she finally received the news of his death on 4 August 1916 during the devastating battle at Pozieres in France.

After the initial shock, Mary's deep grieving galvanised her into action. She decided to follow the example of her women medical colleagues and joined the SWH organisation. Resigning from the Manor Hospital, she obtained a position by December 1916 to serve as a surgeon with Dr Agnes Bennett's America Unit at Ostrovo.

Malta

September–October 1916, Autumn

If the women in this book can be said to be uncommon or atypical, then Dr Eveline Rosetta Benjamin Cohen was especially so. Eveline was the only Tasmanian representative amongst the Australian women doctors who went to war and seems to be the only Australian Jewish woman to serve as a doctor in World War I. Her family were early settlers in Tasmania and Eveline was born in Hobart. After completing her schooling there and wishing to qualify as a doctor, she travelled to Scotland and enrolled at the Edinburgh College of Medicine for Women, beginning her studies in 1905. She won the silver medal for anatomy in her first year and graduated with exceptional results in 1909. Before the war, Eveline was CO and MO for the London Jewish Women's VAD and practised at Hatton Gardens, a narrow commercial street in the heart of London, two blocks from the Thames to the south and Soho to the west.

In the autumn of 1916, Eveline was one of the women doctors who took up the WO's offer of working with the RAMC and on 25 September 1916 she walked up the gangplank of the hospital ship the HMHS *Glengorm Castle* with the ninth group of women doctors to travel overseas with the Women's Medical Unit of the RAMC. She soon joined Irene Eaton in the hospitals in Malta.

By October 1916, Irene and Eveline were at work on the island of Malta when Elsie Dalyell arrived on HMHS *Galeka*. Her journey had begun at Southampton where she had boarded the massive White Star Line ship HMHS *Britannic* off the Isle of Wight on the final day of September 1916. A sister ship of the *Titanic*, with four large funnels and three prominent red crosses along each side, the ship had 3310 beds for patients.[52] The medical personnel's accommodations were the luxuriously furnished cabins of pre-war first-class passengers, and from their cabin portholes and the decks they watched the coast of Portugal pass by, eventually mooring under the lights of Gibraltar. Their route took them past Sardinia and on to Naples for coal, which was 'in the shadow of the cloud-crowned giant Vesuvius'.[53]

Nine hours after passing Mt Etna, the *Britannic* reached the harbour of Mudros on the island of Lemnos, the Allied base for the Dardanelles campaign. The harbour was packed with boats of every kind, from small fishing boats and black cargo boats to hospital ships and the dreadnought battleships of the British navy. This was the point of transshipment for doctors, nurses and VADs going to Malta and they changed to a much smaller and less well-appointed boat, the converted Union-Castle liner the *Galeka*. The ship had just been emptied of soldiers suffering from dysentery and various fevers and was much overloaded. Many of the arriving medical staff on the ship became ill and required medical treatment themselves when they reached the island.[54]

Elsie's trip from Southampton to Malta had taken two weeks of Mediterranean crossing and recrossing but she arrived safely.

Fortune had favoured Elsie's trips twice. Eleven days after she had safely reached Malta, the *Galeka* hit a German mine and sank off Le Havre on the French coast. The boat had once more been en route to Malta and nineteen of the RAMC personnel on board were killed. Then six weeks after Elsie had left the *Britannic* on Mudros, the mighty ship was also sunk by a mine, off the Greek island of Kea, on another trip to Lemnos, and thirty passengers drowned.

Many military hospitals had been established in Salonica by 1916 for soldiers wounded on the Eastern Front, which meant that most necessary surgical treatment had been completed before they arrived in Malta. By the summer and autumn of 1916, when the three Australian women doctors arrived, Malta's hospitals were dealing mainly with malaria, and in the second half of 1916, at least seventy-five per cent of all admissions were for this mosquito-borne illness. Irene and Elsie were involved in the bacteriology of identifying different strains of malaria and dysentery.

In October 1916, Malta's hospitals reached their peak occupancy with 24,750 sick and wounded on the island. Medical staff were not immune from infection of course and in 1917 Dr Isobel Tate from Ireland died of typhoid fever and was buried with full military honours in the Pieta Military Cemetery on 30 January. By 1919, 1303 victims of the war had been buried in the cemetery.

Malta's climate was generally amenable to the soldiers' recovery but from July to September the air on Malta was thick with heat, humidity and dust brought from the south-east by the wind called 'the Sirocco'. The soldier patients, once they were well enough to be out of bed, found their convalescent uniforms, especially the red neckerchiefs, hot and ill-fitting, and the flies were a constant pest. But there were plenty of entertainments and day passes that allowed them to be island tourists for short periods and the flat roofs of the buildings provided cooler places to sit at sunset. Red Cross volunteers brought writing paper, envelopes, cigarettes, butterscotch, chocolate and acid drops to the wards.[55]

For the OCs on Malta, feeding thousands of patients and staff was an endless struggle. Water was scarce in summer, which made getting rid of dust in the wards impossible, and while fresh vegetables and fruit were available on the island, everything else had to be imported. Eggs and chicken, for example, came from Egypt, Tunisia and Italy and the milk was Nestlé's Condensed in tins, which meant it was always sweet.[56] Milk-boys, with their little herds of goats, would stop at houses and hospitals providing milk on-the-hoof into cups or pans to those prepared to try it. Butter was scarce so the soldiers soaked their breakfast toast in milk to make a kind of pudding. The cooked meal of the day was lunch – stew and potatoes with sago, rice or maizena pudding – and later there was beef, tea and cocoa.

In April 1917, when Irene had been on the island for seven months, Eveline for six and Elsie for five, the Malta Garrison received orders to equip and make ready five general hospitals of just over 1000 beds, each to be moved to Salonica. German submarine attacks and mines had made travelling from Salonica to Malta increasingly dangerous. The Aegean was becoming a graveyard for the ships of the British navy and anxious trips were made more so by lifeboat drills and scanning the sea for torpedoes.[57] Malta's Hospitals 61, 62, 63, 64 and 65 were prepared for the move and Elsie went with Hospital No. 63 to Salonica in June 1917. Eveline served on the island until September 1917 and Irene also completed her year's contract with the RAMC.

London, England

Late 1916, Winter

In London, Dr Emma Buckley was the only woman doctor working at the King George Military Hospital, where the laboratory was investigating Malta fever, trench fever and trench nephritis, the last being a nasty inflammation of the kidneys for which neither cause nor cure was unearthed during the war years. Emma knew the enormous hospital well, having been there many times to take samples and tests. The King George was housed in a brand-new building that had been built for His Majesty's Stationery Office and Stores, and an appeal was launched to furnish the wards just after war was declared. Donors could 'buy' a bed for £25 each and 1650 were sold within a fortnight.

The building had tunnels constructed directly underneath, a forward-thinking design intended to enable the delivery of stationery goods and stores directly from Waterloo Station. Instead, the tunnels were first used to bring soldiers from the ambulance trains arriving at Waterloo, providing a smooth transition away from the eyes of the public.

The laboratories where Emma spent more than two years were on the ground floor along with the dispensaries, dining rooms and barracks for 200 orderlies.[58] She wore her khaki uniform with the RAMC's official buttons, but women doctors were not permitted to wear the RAMC badges until 1918, so she wore a King George Hospital badge instead. Emma was unhappy that her rank was not visibly recognised, but pleased that the RAMC had given her a chance to work in a war hospital whereas the AAMC had not.[59]

All of the Australian women doctors who served during the Great War spent time in the heart of the Empire, London – a place of frenetic life and also of suffering and death. Some completed their entire war service in London; some served firstly in London and then other parts of Britain; others served in England and then in France or Serbia or Malta; and a few did not serve in England or London at all, spending their entire war service in places like Belgium, Montenegro and Russia. But all of them came and went through London many times; firstly on arrival, then for recuperation between assignments and to relocate to new positions. They were tourists in London but also part of the strong expatriate Australian community that was well established before the war and then greatly bolstered by it.

London was a powerful magnet for Australians well before World War I.[60] The population of Greater London was a vast 7 million in 1917, ten times more than that of Melbourne and more than Australia's total population of 5 million.[61] World War I served to increase the vibrancy of London, partly because of its proximity to the fighting and partly due to the constant and mammoth movement of people through the capital. The city was the hub of British military administration and most of the 9 million soldiers of the Empire passed through London several times: on their arrival, on periods of leave or for medical treatment.

Australian military and Army Nursing Service headquarters were situated in Horseferry Road, London, although the soldiers called it Cowpunt Road. Soldiers and nurses could pick up their pay and leave passes, obtain new uniforms, store their kit, read Australian newspapers and scan the HQ noticeboards covered with ads for shows, tours and invitations.[62]

The *British Australasian* newspaper was essential reading for soldiers and expats, with its pages of casualty lists but also of new arrivals, the whereabouts of Australians and New Zealanders and social events. The paper also published *The Colonials' Guide to London: For Anzac, Canadian and Other Overseas Visitors.* The immense size and population of the city impressed the Australian visitors and they noted the proximity of both wealth and poverty on the city's streets as well as the amazing technology of tunnels under the Thames, double-decker buses and the Underground railway with its moving staircases.

In a letter to her family in May 1917, Dr Vera Scantlebury wrote:

> My first experience of the tube almost made me ill . . . but [I] find them more convenient than buses . . . The whole arrangement is like a rabbit warren. The air is warm and dank . . . You ascend to the good fresh air, again by a moving staircase. I nearly died the first time. You go upstairs while you are standing still! Now isn't that ridiculous? True![63]

The astonishing increase in the city's transient population had a profound effect on the hotels, restaurants, cafes and entertainments in inner London. As the casualties of war mounted, so did the desire to be entertained and London's clubs, theatres and cinemas were constantly packed. Musicals like *The Bing Boys Are Here*, *Maid of the Mountains* and the *Zig Zag* review were very popular with the soldiers.[64] When Vera's Melbourne University colleagues and her brother Cliff were on leave, they attended the plays and musical productions together and wanted to enjoy every minute of the time they had away from the front. JM Barrie's play *Peter Pan* was a great favourite as well as Australian Oscar Asche's musical comedy *Chu Chin Chow*, based on the tale of Ali Baba, which ran for more than 2000 performances.[65] The stage sets were spectacular, with exotic costumes, unusual dance routines and animals like a camel and a donkey as part of the cast. Sydney doctor Elizabeth Hamilton-Browne and Vera enjoyed the latter together in March 1918.

London's wartime streets were also feverishly busy with the long food queues, the buildings plastered with recruitment and war bond posters, and the famous monuments mostly sandbagged. Vera wrote of the unreality of being out for dinner in a place full of people and music with the war going on just across the English Channel.[66] After dining with a Melbourne friend at the Piccadilly Grill Room she wrote of the strangeness of all the lights and gaiety in such a terrible time yet also that it was good to forget for a little while. She had experienced a very worrying time in her wards at the Endell Street Military Hospital that morning.[67]

While German Zeppelin airships had intermittently dropped bombs on London since January 1915, from the spring of 1917 there were new and more deadly threats from air-raids. The first raid to use conventional aircraft was in May 1917 when twenty-three Gotha bombers dropped more than 100 bombs, killing seventy-one people and causing panic in East London.[68] Endell Street Military Hospital was close to the areas targeted by the bombings and in September 1917 shrapnel fell on the building but caused no physical injuries:

> The noise was terrific but more melodious than before when we only heard the sickening thud and crash of falling bombs. The shriek of the shells from our guns as they passed through the air made a moaning sound, then there came the explosions of the shells and the shuddering noise of the guns . . . then a sudden expectant lull when all seemed so still in the moonlight and in this lull the strains of the harmonium from the recreation room became louder and the men still singing songs.[69]

The women doctors and nurses at Endell Street felt that they had to display calm and assurance during the raids as many of the men were immobilised and could not be moved, and for some, the bombing was a reminder of the trenches. Vera even considered putting herself into the Thomas splint used for fractured femurs to experience what it felt like to be unable to move in the presence of danger.

Australia's expatriate community in London was bolstered from early 1915 by the arrival of Australian families and women who made their way to England to be closer to their enlisted sons and husbands, and to make their own contribution to the war effort.[70] Some middle- and upper-class Australian families created comfortable homes in central London flats, replete with a family matriarch and English domestic servants.[71] For example, Melbourne woman Mary Bage, who had lost her son Captain Robert Bage when he was killed on the Gallipoli Peninsula in May 1915, arrived in London with her daughter Ethel in 1916. Perhaps proximity to the war zone may have allowed Mary to feel closer to her lost son and it gave her some comfort to provide for others as she had not been able to provide for him. Ethel worked at the London Red Cross office for prisoners of war and Mary's niece Jessie was a VAD nurse in England and France.[72]

Women like Mary Bage provided a family atmosphere for their many young Australian visitors. They hosted dinners and social events, inviting interesting guests and providing welcome distraction for young doctors like Vera Scantlebury and Rachel Champion. At Mary's flat, for example, they talked with writer Stella Miles Franklin, who had just returned from Macedonia where she worked as an orderly with the SWH under another Victorian doctor, Mary De Garis. Sir Douglas Mawson and his wife Paquita were regular visitors too. Mary Bage's son had been a member of Mawson's 1911–1914 Antarctic Expedition as was the photographer Frank Hurley, whose World War I photographic exhibition at London's Grafton Gallery in April 1918 was visited by many Australian expatriates. Despite the close Australian community in London, Vera wrote, 'Homesickness is one of the worst maladies.'[73]

Part 4

1917

Chapter 5

'The brightest link in our love-chain broken'

About 2 am Sunday began the hurricane; by 3 am most
of the Unit was up endeavouring to save the tents from
collapsing. By 8 am practically every tent in the hospital had
collapsed . . . The tent stores (groceries, linen, splints etc)
were scattered abroad. The X-ray and dark room tents were
both in ribbons. Such a scene of desolation.[1]

Dr Mary De Garis, Macedonia, 1918

Eastern Front: Russia

January 1917, Winter
In early March 1917 a telegram from Galicia arrived at the
SWH headquarters in Edinburgh bearing the tragic news that
Dr Laura Forster had died: 'Doctor Forster Died typhoid
Zaleschiki January Twenty Nine Russian particulars.' The
telegram was addressed to Dr Beatrice Russell, the Chair of
the Personnel Committee of the SWH. A colleague, Dr Alice
Benham, who had served with Laura in Belgium during the
first weeks of war, described her as 'a fair woman with an

indomitable courage, and a love of adventure, which led her into many out-of-the-way corners of the world.'[2]

Laura Forster had travelled thousands of kilometres since her service in Belgium and France in the first months of the war in 1914 and 1915. She was happy to travel independently to wherever she believed her medical skills could be used. Having arrived in the city of Petrograd in the winter of 1915 and working initially in a large men's hospital – a medical taboo pre-war – she moved to the nearby NUWSS maternity hospital in April 1916 but continued her surgical work at the men's hospital whenever there was time. In June 1916, she joined a Russian Red Cross unit that was headed by a leading Russian woman surgeon. They were bound for the Caucasus in southern Russia.[3]

Two years earlier, in April 1914, Russia had attempted to regain land lost in the Russo–Turkish War of the late 1880s, causing war to erupt between the Russian and Ottoman Empires. The lands of the South Caucasus today include Armenia, southern Azerbaijan and southern Georgia, between the Black Sea and the Caspian Sea, and this was the area where the battles raged from 1914 to early 1917. By mid-1915, the countryside was flooded with tens of thousands of Armenian refugees fleeing the genocide by the Ottoman Empire and thousands more displaced by the battles all along the Russian–Ottoman border area.

In wartime, the Russian Society of the Red Cross (RSRC) was the umbrella organisation for the allocation of all medical resources and provided the Third Advance Squadron medical unit for the battles in the Caucasus.[4] The RSRC had opened hospitals near the frontlines and established hundreds of infirmaries, soup kitchens and evacuation centres as well as transporting the wounded.

By April 1916 the Russian army had advanced as far as Erzurum in eastern Turkey and the ancient port of Trabzon along the Turkish northern coast. Between June and September 1916, Russian casualties were at least 50,000, the majority dying from illness. Laura worked somewhere in this maelstrom of wounded and sick soldiers and refugees in Erzurum and found the heat and dust of the 1916 summer difficult to cope with. In August, ill and worn out, she cabled the NUWSS from Tiflis (now Tbilisi, Georgia) some 600 kilometres north-east of Erzurum to say that she was finding conditions there intolerable and would like to return to a NUWSS unit in Russia.

The NUWSS posted her to a Millicent Fawcett Hospital unit in Kazan, deep in south-west Russia. Dr Alice Benham, Laura's colleague from her time in Belgium in 1914, was in charge of a hospital for refugees in Stara Chelnoe, near Kazan, and needed to return to England. Laura travelled the 2000 kilometres to Kazan and took over the little hospital for three months.

In December 1916, Dr King-Atkinson, CO of another NUWSS hospital in Galicia, heard that her husband had been wounded in France and wanted to return to England. Laura again travelled more than 2000 kilometres, this time to the west, to reach Zaleschiki (Zalishchyky, Ukraine) and take charge of the 52nd Epidemic Hospital there. Australian Florence MacDowell, who had also joined the Millicent Fawcett Hospital units, was the matron of this eighty-bed hospital in a huge building with patients suffering from scarlet fever, influenza, dysentery, typhoid and a range of other infectious diseases.[5]

Wherever the women doctors and nurses went in Russia and Turkey, they were met with intense curiosity and a barrage of questions about their ages, salaries, husbands and how their wrist-watches worked.

Zaleschiki had been taken and retaken by opposing forces five times since the beginning of the war and was ruined and desolate.

Wounded soldiers, pregnant women, sick children including orphans, and villagers with infectious diseases all flocked to the hospital in Zaleschiki.[6] When Laura arrived there in late 1916, she was fifty-nine years old, very thin and exhausted. She had been travelling and working in challenging conditions continuously for at least eighteen months and, in a weakened state, she contracted typhus. Her heart could not take the strain any longer. Laura was buried in January 1917 with the full funeral rites of the Russian Orthodox Church. Long lines of nurses, nuns and villagers walked through the snow accompanying her final trip, a Union Jack was draped over the coffin and a Russian icon headed the procession.

Greatly beloved by the nurses at Zaleschiki, and everywhere she had worked, Laura's initial experience as a nurse gave her a unique insight into the nurses' point of view and she was always able to win their respect and liking. Her tragic death caused great sorrow both to the NUWSS and SWH communities.

Eastern Front: Northern Macedonia

February 1917, Winter
Dr Agnes Bennett's letters vividly describe the paradoxical experiences of life in the Ostrovo tent hospital. On Boxing Day 1916, she wrote: 'The ground here is covered in the sweetest little mauve crocuses – tiny things.'[7] But a month later on 23 January 1917, her thoughts are more sombre when she writes, 'The horrible mortality that comes of these long rough journeys in the ambulances – we had 9 arrived here dead.'[8]

Dr Mary De Garis, who arrived the following month, was also taken by the beauty of the lake and mountains around the camp. After taking the train to Southampton and then a steamship through the Mediterranean to Salonica, Mary was warmly welcomed by Agnes Bennett and a very rough car ride north to the SWH's Ostrovo hospital in northern Macedonia. She had been appointed as second in charge under Dr Bennett.

Her life as a surgeon began in earnest when, in her first month, she was sent up to the dressing station at Dobraveni to give Dr Lilian Cooper a much-needed break. The camp had just been moved and Mary was sent to supervise. She managed to conceal the extent of her ignorance, which included being unaware that all the tents should be trenched to prevent flooding in a downpour. By observing people and occasionally making useful suggestions, Mary acquired credit for a profundity of practical knowledge she did not really have.[9]

Dobraveni, halfway up one of the foothills of the Voras Mountains, was a desolate, windswept and treeless place. But Mary found the social life interesting and the constant air-raids added a 'spice of excitement'; their system of 'funk holes' (trenches) helped to shelter them effectively. [10]

The hospital camp at Ostrovo presented constant challenges to the chief medical officers. Agnes and Mary were responsible for the welfare of around 250 people and were consequently very particular about the sanitation as the camp was not sewered; there were copious flies and wasps, and mosquito-borne malaria was endemic in the area and across the Eastern Front. This meant preparation and care of the camp's latrines and urinals was vital in minimising outbreaks of dysentery and highly infectious diar-rhoea, which was especially dangerous to recovering patients. The latrines were constantly filled in and a record was kept of the position of the sites that had already been used.

To battle malaria, Mary ordered that the nearby swamp be drained. Staff tried to cover up as much as possible, wearing gaiters and using mosquito nets, particularly after dark. At the first sign of a high temperature, the doctors administered quinine injections, which they had found to be the most effective treatment. The staff, however, dreaded the painful intramuscular injections that were administered with long needles.

Agnes and Mary were also required to adhere to the Serbian army's military rules for camp discipline, managing the complexities of patient administration with the Serbian army and issues of staff administration with the SWH. They dealt therefore with a huge range of medical and morale issues, including camp food, provisions, equipment, accommodation, sanitation, personalities, the Serbian male helpers and even the cultivation of the vegetables.[11] Mary's brother Jack sent boxes of Australian dried fruit from the family business in Mildura, which were very much appreciated by the staff.

Surgery was a daily challenge at both the dressing station at Dobraveni and the Ostrovo hospital. Agnes recounted a story of Mary's surgical work with Nurses Angell and Saunders, who were operating in a tent at the dressing station. An air-raid had begun and bombs were dropping around them, but Mary steadily worked to extract a bullet from the palate of a French soldier. They carried on calmly like a well-oiled machine:

> There were fifteen aeroplanes aiming at them, and the camp next to them, which suffered very badly. The women's presence of mind and courage during air-raids and bombardments have been a source of amazement and admiration to me . . . Only those who know what it is to have bombs falling all round them can realise what an amount of presence of mind and courage such a thing takes.[12]

The surgical work performed at Ostrovo was impressive even when it ebbed and flowed depending on the battles that raged over the mountains just beyond the hospital. In the three years from September 1916 to October 1919, the estimated number of surgical procedures performed was 1084. These included eighty amputations, mostly of fingers and toes, twelve re-amputations, thirty-eight bomb wounds, eighteen bullet wounds, twenty-six compound fractures, ninety hernias, eighty removals of foreign bodies, thirty shrapnel wounds, twenty-four curettage of old wounds and 390 repairing and scraping of old wounds. Over this period, 103 patients died.[13] The workload was often relentless, exhausting and distressing and required extraordinary resilience.

Mary wrote about her cases and provided a unique snapshot of five patients in her ward:

> two Serbs (one a plating of a leg, the other a wound of hand), one Frenchman (operated for appendicitis); a Turk (with both eyeballs excised and injury to the hand) and a Canadian (both of whose hips had been dislocated).[14]

She was very proud of how she and Dr Jean Rose, a newly qualified Scottish graduate who had recently arrived, successfully treated the Canadian who had been thrown from a cart in an accident, dislocating both hips. They anaesthetised him, made their diagnosis, laid him on the floor of the tent then, with one on each side, the doctors manually manipulated his hips back into place and encased one side in plaster after X-rays were taken. The soldier stayed for eight weeks of recovery and was very popular with the Serbian patients.[15]

The autumn of 1917 saw staff changes as the exhausted Lilian Cooper and Josephine Bedford left in September. In Lilian's eight months of service 152 patients were admitted and she performed 144 operations.[16] She experienced recurring bronchitis and by mid-August 1917, had developed pneumonia. Lilian and Josephine decided to recuperate in London and then return home to the warmth of Brisbane. For her bravery the Serbian Crown Prince awarded Lilian Cooper the Medal of St Sava, 4th Class, and Josephine Bedford the Medal of St Sava, 5th Class.[17]

The following month, Agnes Bennett became very ill with malaria while up at Dobraveni and, on her return by ambulance to Ostrovo, the staff were horrified by her colour and debility. After sixteen months as CMO, twelve near the frontline, Agnes reluctantly resigned and, after warm but exhausting farewell dinners with the Serbians, her staff and patients, she was transported by car to board a ship at Salonica and return home via Cairo to recuperate. In Cairo, Agnes received the news that her brother Bob, 'that splendid boy' she had met up with in Alexandria over a year earlier, had been killed in the murderous Battle of Passchendaele. Grief-stricken and missing her family terribly, she joined the troopship HMAT *Wiltshire* as a medical officer and sailed home to Sydney.[18]

Mary De Garis was appointed as her successor and took command of the Ostrovo hospital. Camp life continued on with a variety of contrasting personalities and experiences. Musical evenings, theatricals and dinners relieved the stress and boredom. Often the festivities would close with the Serbian national folk dance, the *kola*. Many of the women learned the dance and Mary loved to join in.

There were many humorous moments, as some of the patients and staff, such as the writer Stella Miles Franklin, were very entertaining. Appointed as a volunteer cook and orderly, Miles arrived in September 1917 and wrote witty observations of camp life. She called the dreaded quinine injections 'bayonet charges' and wrote: 'It was said that on coming to Macedonia one lost her hair during the first year, her teeth during the second and her character during the third.'[19]

Like most of the SWH staff, Mary suffered from serious illnesses during her nineteen months in Macedonia, including typhoid, dysentery and malaria. Emotionally, she was in deep mourning for Colin Thomson but sublimated her grief in her work at the hospital.[20] Her energy and dedication were legendary.

Mary's leadership was evident on a wintry February night in 1918. At around 3 am, after heavy snowfalls and rain, a hurricane blew for about six hours, virtually demolishing the entire hospital. Only three of the seventy tents were left upright. Precious medical supplies were scattered and equipment broken. The patients had to be rescued from the collapsed tents in high winds and driving rain by staff who had crawled out from under their own tents dressed in their pyjamas. All but seventeen of the patients were then evacuated by train to other hospitals.

Working frantically, Mary, the Serbian male helpers (*bolnichars*) and staff had the main tents repaired and re-erected and 100 beds ready for patients by the end of the week. Mary wrote to the SWH administrators:

It was really sad to see our beautiful comfortable camp, of which we were all so proud, such a wreck . . . we are all proud to say that we admitted five patients this morning – we were not *quite* ready for them, but we managed, and tonight we are ready for twenty more, and are a real hospital again . . . In fact, I am proud of my Unit, and think you will be the same. Mary De Garis.[21]

They were extremely lucky that no fires had broken out as there were charcoal burners in every tent. The following week, a new shipment of tents and medical equipment arrived fortuitously, having been ordered months previously by Mary to guard against such emergencies.[22]

Dover, England

January–May 1917, Autumn

In England, Dr Katie Ardill had been at work at the County of Middlesex War Hospital in Napsbury for ten months when she was transferred to Dover Military Hospital in January 1917. The Kent coastline from Dover to Hythe was of vital strategic importance to the Allies, and millions of soldiers and other personnel passed through the ports of Dover and Folkestone between 1914 and 1919.

On 27 August 1914, the regular afternoon boat from Boulogne to Folkestone had brought the first sad collection of British wounded to England. Boulogne in France became the principal port for embarkation of Allied wounded throughout the war and Dover and Folkestone, the main ports where the wounded were brought home. During the war years, Dover dealt with 1,260,506 casualties, unloaded more than 4000 boats full of wounded, then loaded patients into the twenty ambulance trains or the single emergency train for dangerously wounded.

The hospital sat several levels above Dover Harbour, with its incessant activity of troop and hospital ships. Katie had a clear view of the panorama from the hospital's windows, which included Dover Castle, its massive grey walls atop the famous white chalk cliffs being the last sight of England for soldiers going to war and their first on returning.

The hospital's patients included soldiers like 21-year-old Gunner Alec Sim.[23] Alec was a farmer from Lake Bolac in Victoria who joined the 3rd Australian Field Artillery Brigade and arrived in England the same month Katie arrived in Dover – January 1917. A gas attack delivered by German aircraft at Passchendaele in France poisoned his lungs on 3 June that year and left him dangerously ill.

Many different types of gases were used by both sides in World War I but the gases that brought terrible suffocation were phosgene and chloropicrin. Phosgene caused little irritation when it floated across the ground and soldiers were often gassed before they were aware of being exposed. Chloropicrin was frequently added to phosgene because its immediate irritating effect caused violent coughing and vomiting and tended to delay or prevent the wearing of a gas mask, allowing the phosgene to do its insidious work.[24] Oxygen through a mask was the most effective treatment for serious cases but when a gassed soldier collapsed or was unconscious, an apparatus with a foot pump that fed a face mask through a portable tube was attempted.

Alec was transferred urgently to England on HMHS *Stad Antwerpen*. He died at 7.40 pm on 7 June 1917 when his heart could not cope with the struggle to breathe, his lungs fatally damaged. Alec was given a military funeral; his coffin was draped with the Union Jack and carried by gun carriage to the graveyard. A funeral service, firing party and bugler farewelled him. He was buried in a grave in St James' Churchyard Cemetery, Dover, in a coffin of fine polished elm. The Sim family received a full burial report and a sealed parcel containing Alec's personal items, such as letters, photos, his watch and pocket knife and a broken fountain pen. Their tribute said that Alec was 'The brightest link in our love-chain broken'.[25]

London, England

March 1917, Spring

Queenslander Dr Mabel Murray-Prior had completed three years of her medical degree in Sydney when she arrived in London in early 1915. After a year of working as a VAD she completed her medical qualification in Dublin and her MD in Edinburgh in 1917. She was appointed to the Royal Herbert Hospital near Greenwich in London. The hospital was dedicated to the recuperation and rehabilitation of wounded soldiers.When Mabel arrived at the Royal Herbert, a hospital built for the veterans of the Crimean War, she found a distinctive kind of recuperative environment. The building was based on a revolutionary pavilion design much influenced by the nursing principles of Florence Nightingale. The wards were separate wings connected to a central corridor and designed to maximise sunlight and fresh air intake on each side of the rows of beds. A large arched floor-to-ceiling window at the end of each ward meant that patients could look out over the 7 hectares of hilltop parkland.[26]

Arriving by hospital train, the soldier patients were met at nearby Woolwich Station by VADs waiting at long wooden trestle tables with mugs of every size and kettles on the boil. Those able to walk left the train first. A VAD at the hospital and writer, Enid Bagnold, described the scene:

> The station entrance is full of men crowding in and taking the steaming mugs of tea and coffee; men on pickaback [sic] with bandaged feet; men with only a nose and one eye showing, with stumbling legs, bound arms. The station, for five minutes, is full of jokes and witticisms; then they pass out and into the waiting chars-à-bancs [sic].[27]

Across the parkland was the extensive Greenwich Cemetery where, during the war years, 558 soldiers from the Royal Herbert and the nearby Brook War Hospital were buried. When a soldier died on Mabel's wards, orderlies arrived carrying a stretcher and a folded Union Jack flag. Behind the screens placed around the bed, his body was covered with the flag and was then carried out through the ward. Every patient who was able to, stood to attention.

It was the Australian flag that draped the body of 38-year-old AAMC doctor Captain Ronald Lennox Henderson as he was carried out of a ward at the Royal Herbert. Like Mabel, he came from Queensland and was a regimental MO with the 2nd Australian General Hospital at Wimereux in France. Ronald had received a gunshot wound to the head while caring for wounded soldiers under heavy fire, an action for which he was given a Military Cross. Other than operating to relieve the pressure in his skull, there was little that Mabel or any of the doctors on staff could do. His medical record shows that he had a large number of foreign bodies in his brain and he never regained consciousness, dying on the last day of July 1917. He was buried at Brookwood Military Cemetery with a firing party of 120 buglers.[28]

These were the tragedies that Mabel witnessed often and, being a vivacious and warm-hearted woman, the deaths must have been gruelling. Enid Bagnold wrote that death was such a constant companion that she was 'afraid of waking up and finding it commonplace'.[29] After six months, Mabel was transferred to the Edinburgh Hospital, which was in urgent need of more medical staff.

London, England

March 1917, Spring

Back in Melbourne, Dr Vera Scantlebury bid her final farewells to her family on 14 February 1917 as the HMTS *Morea* moved away from the Port Melbourne pier. The paper streamers in their hands finally snapped; she called it 'our day of waving goodbye and breaking ribbons'.[30] Vera was twenty-seven years old and her father really did not want her to go; she was the Senior Medical Officer (SMO) at Melbourne's Children's Hospital, the first woman to hold a senior residency, and she had just become unofficially engaged.

Forty-two women had completed a medical degree at the University of Melbourne when Vera enrolled in 1907 and of the fifty-seven students in her final-year class in 1913 only four were women. In her first professional appointment as a junior resident at the Melbourne Hospital in 1914, she was the only woman of the eighteen appointments.

Despite her family's concerns, Vera was determined to serve and obtained a position as an assistant surgeon at the Endell Street Military Hospital in London where her Melbourne University friend Dr Rachel Champion was already at work. The cablegram in October 1916 from Dr Flora Murray, Endell Street's co-founder, read: 'Appointment military hospital Endell St certain May first passage unpaid cable if not accepted Murray.'[31]

Also being farewelled on that February day were soldiers heading to Deir el Belah, 20 kilometres southwest of Gaza in Palestine as reinforcements of the Australian Light Horse.[32] When the boat reached Adelaide, Dr Phoebe Chapple joined Vera on board the *Morea*. Phoebe was on her way to England with the intention of joining the SWH.[33] Many Australians on their way to war felt like tourists during the boat trip; this was especially so for the women doctors who generally travelled in shared first- or second-class cabins or as ship's doctors. Being unable to officially enlist, they paid their own way; the *Morea*'s fare for Vera was £129, roughly valued at $A10,300 today and equivalent to about forty-five weeks of the average male salary in 1914.

The first record of Vera's travels begins with her being rowed ashore in Port Said.[34] She was 'stoney broke' so could do little but hire an 'Arabia', a horse-drawn carriage, from which to admire the wide boulevards, deep verandahs and street cafes with her colleague Phoebe Chapple. Vera sketched the headwear of 'two well veiled Mohomedan [sic] women'[35] showing a tiny cotton-reel arrangement between their eyes. She and Phoebe had their fortunes told in the hope that the whereabouts of German submarines might be predicted.

Vera and Phoebe's boat passed through the Strait of Messina just five months after Dr Elsie Dalyell had travelled in the opposite direction on her way to Malta. The *Morea* reached the port of Marseilles in France on 30 March 1917, six weeks after leaving Melbourne, and Vera and Phoebe packed in readiness for the cross-country train trip to Boulogne on the north-west coastline of France, to be followed by a boat to England. Their train rattled through Paris during the night but at Amiens 'we heard the guns being fired then we passed into the war zone about 15–30 miles behind the frontier'.[36] On one of the stations a poster suggested:

> A wise old owl sat on an oak
> The more he saw, the less he spoke
> The less he spoke, the more he heard
> Soldiers should imitate this wise bird.

At Boulogne, a bitter wind, hail and sleet made Vera's search for the 13th Stationary Hospital a trial. Her younger brother Cliff, also a doctor, was thought to be with the 13th but to her intense disappointment, she found he had been transferred to the No. 49 Casualty Clearing Station, which had been moved on the previous week.

Once in London, Phoebe stayed only long enough to be posted by the RAMC to the Cambridge Military Hospital in Aldershot, 80 kilometres to the south-west of London. Vera took up lodgings at 25 Wimpole Street, the home of Endell Street Military Hospital's ear, nose and throat specialist Dr Octavia Lewin, and enjoyed her bed-sitting room on the top floor of the house. At both the hospital and Wimpole Street she was immersed in suffragist communities and, like her Queensland colleague Dr Eleanor Bourne, was sometimes impatient with the constant discussion of 'the vote'.

The OCs, Doctors Murray and Garrett Anderson, were well aware that the pace, intensity, smell and sheer awfulness of military surgery was confronting to newly appointed surgeons, especially those as young and inexperienced as Doctors Scantlebury and Champion. They frequently offered the staff respite by making their comfortable cottage at Penn in the countryside of Buckinghamshire available. They also initially gave newcomers the responsibility for only one ward, less complex surgical procedures and practice in the application of anaesthetics, which allowed for observation of surgery.

During the war there were essentially four types of general anaesthetics: chloroform and ether, and for shorter surgeries, ethyl chloride or a mixture of nitrous oxide and oxygen. There was novocaine for local anaesthesia and stovain for operations on the pelvis or legs. There were also several methods of application but a combination often used was to begin with chloroform, given slowly by the drop method, onto a mask with a single layer of gauze. This was followed by ether, also dropped slowly onto a second mask with two layers of gauze.[37] Vera's diary letters reveal that during her first five weeks at the hospital, she was mostly acting as an anaesthetist and administering chloroform.[38] On 5 June 1917, in her fifth week at the hospital, she sent men into the 'land of nod' between 2 pm and 8.30 pm but also completed her first operation on a soldier's arm.[39]

Vera's surviving diary letters provide one of the few original sources of insight into doctors' emotional responses to their surgical work during the war. The work was physically and psychologically tough and the soldiers' wounds were often 'multiple and of a truly "shocking" nature'.[40]

Vera had barely three years of hospital experience and said in an early letter, 'This work is so entirely different from anything I have ever done – I am so slow in brain and body.'[41] She knew immediately that her knowledge of anatomy was inadequate for the technical demands of military surgery and coped at first by studying her university anatomy textbook at night. Later she practised her technique in the anatomy dissection room of the LSMW.[42]

During her early days at the hospital Vera wrote of her attempts to handle two gunshot wounds: 'Opened and drained wound – Did it badly – clumsy – fingers all thumbs. Practically told so by CO.' In late June 1917 she wrote:

I am not at all keen on military surgery but I shall get used to it and do it better than at pres. But I think it is horrible . . . It is so awful to struggle along when you are only half-hearted – the wounds are so awful.[43]

But by October she told her family, 'I did five ops yesterday, they are still alive today which is something . . . I am liking the work better although some fractures nearly drive me mad.'[44] After nine months of surgery, on a dark day of intense cold in January 1917, she performed four of the day's nineteen operations: 'Two amputations, a hunt for the muscular spinal nerve which I found and released it from an obnoxious adhesion which was binding it so tightly it could not do its work.'[45]

Her letters portray her transition from self-doubt and a lack of confidence to a feeling of relative competence. It is a journey that many surgeons, both male and female, would have experienced during the war.

Alongside the surgical cases were men suffering from the appalling effects of gas poisoning and from pneumonia, pleurisy and malaria. War did not exempt soldiers from suffering from everyday problems either, such as hernias, gastric ulcers, cardiac disease and rheumatism, sometimes in combination with their wounds.

On a typical day for Vera and the other Australian women doctors in London during 1917 – Eleanor Bourne, Elizabeth Hamilton-Browne, Rachel Champion and Emma Buckley – they would often begin with letter-writing before breakfast.[46] By 9 am they would be attending 'the rag' at Endell Street, where Dr Garrett Anderson joined the surgeons, pathologist and matron to hear the overnight report from the orderly officer. The surgeons took their turn every fortnight to act as the orderly officer, which meant being in charge of the hospital overnight and sleeping there, although their sleep was often interrupted as convoys arrived at all times of the night.

The scene in the hospital courtyard was rather impressive. It was very early morning and not quite dark. The ambulance girls and stretcher bearers were lined up waiting on one side and the night sister stood on the other with her lantern – The Sargeant Major (a man!) dodged about. Then came the ambulances. Silently the stretchers were lifted down from the motors which held four and a nurse – I had a great feeling of pity, a fellow feeling.[47]

Morning ward rounds were followed by wound dressings. Lunchtime provided a chance for a break away from the hospital and sometimes they might lunch at the Regent Palace Hotel, a favourite place with Australians, before afternoon surgery commenced. Vera described the operating theatre as

that beehive . . . with its hot stifling atmosphere and white gowned and hooded women moving ceaselessly about and stretchers pushed hither and thither and the sweet heavy sickly fumes of the chloroform.[48]

One group of friends who called on the women doctors in London were their male university medical colleagues from home. They visited while on leave from RAMC units in France or when recuperating from wounds. Endell Street Military Hospital was a convenient place of contact and the number of male callers did not go unnoticed. When an Australian naval officer arrived to see Vera in February 1918, an orderly commented, 'not only does she know all the Australian army, now the navy is coming!'[49]

At the end of her very first day at Endell Street, Vera was a little chagrined to find that Captain (Dr) Norman Bullen, a university and Melbourne Hospital colleague, had called at the hospital to enquire after her.[50] They went to lunch the following day, enjoying wine and coffee, and she was sufficiently impressed by the coffee-making machine to sketch it for her family. Sadly, Norman returned to France shortly after but died of wounds on 10 October 1917 during the Third Battle of Ypres.[51] Over the course of the war, Vera and Rachel Champion lost seven of the male colleagues who appeared in a photo taken of them all during their final year of medicine at the University of Melbourne in 1913.

Aldershot, England

March 1917, Spring
When Phoebe Chapple achieved her matriculation certificate in 1895 and, as one of the top students in the state, was awarded a University of Adelaide scholarship, she was sixteen years old. This was considered to be too young to pursue her chosen area of study: medicine. Instead, like Dr Agnes Bennett, she initially completed a degree in science in 1898 before taking her medical degree, achieving second or third place in each year of her course.[52] Phoebe graduated in 1904 and before leaving for England was conducting her medical practice from Prince Alfred College, where her father was Headmaster and the Chapple family lived.

Her approach to the AAMC to enlist in 1914 was rebuffed, but by the summer of 1916, battles like that of the Somme, with almost 60,000 casualties on the first day alone, were applying enormous pressure to medical staff. During that year Adelaide newspapers carried stories of a scarcity of doctors as well as stories of women doctors working in military hospitals and, with the support of her parents, Phoebe decided it was time to offer her services in England.[53]

She boarded HMTS *Morea* in mid-February 1917 at Port Adelaide. On board she was welcomed by Dr Vera Scantlebury, who was ten years younger, and in Phoebe had found an excellent travelling companion.

The women enjoyed day sojourns together at Port Said and Marseilles, and Vera described the snow-clad Mt Etna, seen as their boat traversed the Strait of Messina, as being inexpressibly beautiful. As they approached Marseilles in early April, the Notre Dame Cathedral looked over them from the highest pinnacle above the city. On the cart ride up to visit the church, Phoebe took pity on the thin horse and got out and walked.

Phoebe arrived in Folkestone after a Channel crossing from Boulogne, France, on 7 April 1917 and, once in London, was immediately offered work by the RAMC with the nominal rank of captain. She began in the surgical wards of Cambridge Military Hospital in Aldershot, Hampshire, working with soldiers with many different war wounds and illnesses. The hospital had been the first base hospital in England to receive battle casualties directly from the Western Front and was also the first in England to open a dedicated plastic surgery department for facial wounds. Dr Harold Gillies, considered to be the father of plastic surgery in Britain, began his extraordinary pioneering work there, attempting to give some hope to men whose faces had been terribly damaged by shot and shrapnel.

Cambridge Military Hospital was built on a hill so that the wind might sweep away infections, and the enormous building was crowned by a central five-tiered clock tower with an impressive wind vane. One of the clock tower's three bells was a war trophy captured at Sebastopol during the Crimean War but the bells were not rung in Phoebe's time because the cacophony disturbed the patients' rest. She valued her work at Aldershot as a tremendous experience, adapting quickly to the frenetic pace of the hospital, which accommodated 1000 patients and accepted convoys of sick and wounded from France constantly.[54] In November 1917, after eight months at Aldershot, Phoebe was transferred to the WAAC, promoted to the nominal rank of major and sent to France.

The WAAC was created in the spring of 1917 after the Director General of National Service suggested that he could not find enough men for the firing line unless women could take the place of men in supportive roles.[55] The corps was initially looking for 12,000 women for service in France and an unlimited number in Britain. When recruiting was advertised in the press in late February 1917, the response from women was immediately enthusiastic and thousands came forward. But the head of the new WAAC, Helen Gwynne-Vaughan, an English medical bacteriologist, struggled to recruit enough officers to conduct the enlistment process for so many keen volunteers. The arrival from overseas of doctors like Phoebe Chapple was fortuitous.

The WAAC was quickly organised into companies. A Companies took over from soldiers the cooking, cleaning and laundering of army camps and military hospitals. Part of Phoebe's role would be to check on the health of corps members in A Companies who might have contact with infection in the hospitals. B Companies were clerks, typists, telegraphers and telephonists. C and D Companies were all those employed outside camps, such as bakers, drivers, gardeners and motor mechanics. WAAC personnel essentially took over the kitchens, bakeries and dining rooms in camps and hospitals and prepared food en masse, including savoury rice, fish kedgeree, liver and onions, stews, curries and puddings. The WO estimated that men in the frontline needed 4600 calories a day, which was more than most ate at home previously and often also of better quality.[56]

In the British military camps in France, accommodation for WAAC members varied. Medical officers like Phoebe were frequently on the move between military bases and stayed in many types of accommodation. Some corps women were housed in demountable wooden buildings, some in semi-circular Nissen-type huts and others were billeted in cottages nearby. Their accommodation was often very basic and the lack of even simple hooks and shelves meant that the women often had only their suitcases for storage. A typical day's menu might be: breakfast – boiled bacon, bread, butter, marmalade and tea; dinner – beef stew and a few vegetables, boiled rice and jam for pudding; supper – soup and biscuits or sardines.[57] But the pay was good, with uniform, quarters and rations provided.

From its beginnings in 1917, the WAAC received unwarranted criticism and rumour concerning the members' behaviour, and their right to wear uniform and to adopt military titles. The participation of women wearing khaki and serving near the battle-field upset existing social conventions, and jokes and innuendo were ways to denigrate their work. By April 1918, their work over the previous twelve months during heavy fighting on the Western Front, would be recognised, and Queen Mary of Britain became their Commander in Chief. The WAAC was renamed Queen Mary's Army Auxiliary Corps (QMAAC).

Phoebe's role as a corps doctor was to evaluate corps members on enlistment, monitor their health during their service, and check the sanitation and general suitability of their accommodation and work situations. Phoebe believed that the women in the corps answered every emergency that called them when things looked very bad on the Western Front in 1917 and that although not meant to go into the firing lines, the women were exposed to more danger than was ever intended. Bombs were dropped everywhere, especially during the Battle of the Somme in 1918, and casualties occurred, but corps members continued to work long hours, often at hard physical tasks, without slacking.[58]

Eastern Front: Salonica, Greece

June 1917, Summer

Meanwhile, Dr Elsie Dalyell had travelled from Malta with the No. 63 Hospital to re-establish the unit in Greece, about 12 kilometres north-west of Salonica in the Derveni Pass. Here, the low hills surrounding the hospital were bare and the landscape uninviting, with none of the colour, lively atmosphere and sea breezes of the island of Malta. It was a hospital under canvas with dozens of wards in 18-metre-long marquees with removable sides, essential in the summer when the heat was stifling and it was only possible to work in the early mornings or late evenings. Winter was intensely cold and Elsie would make a 'wigwam' in her tent, which she thought could be mistaken for the mound of a wandering bush turkey.[59]

The hospital's isolation indicates that it was primarily an infectious diseases hospital, as malaria was the greatest enemy to soldiers on both sides along the Salonica Front. Since mosquitoes recognised no boundaries, their elimination would have required cooperation between warring parties, which was not possible. Only late in the war was it understood that preventive measures were possible and preferable, but when malaria reached its peak from July to November in 1916 and 1917 doctors were struggling against this nefarious adversary. In Malta, Elsie's duties had been split between clinical work and pathology but in Salonica she was in charge of the laboratory of the 63rd's 1000-bed hospital.

Malaria was the fourth pathological foe that Elsie had tackled in the laboratory. In Uskub in Serbia it was typhus, in England it was dysentery, at Royaumont in France it had been gas gangrene, and in Salonica it was malaria. Armies on both sides were severely debilitated by malaria, which causes lethargy, fever, headaches and vomiting. In the most severe cases it can cause seizures and comas, and can sometimes be deadly. Elsie diagnosed the fever and distinguished between its different types by examining blood under the microscope using blood films. But the inconsistent supply of the anti-malaria drugs – cinchona bark and quinine – made treatment unreliable, and when soldiers were not properly treated, some would have recurrences of the disease months later.

Elsie was not satisfied with the arrangements for blood transfusion in the camp's hospital and put together improved equipment from the scant apparatus she scrounged from supplies.[60] Both blood transfusion and grouping underwent development during the war and their availability varied across both the Western and Eastern Fronts. Despite the lack of facilities, Elsie's laboratory and her work were impressive.

London, England

October 1917, Autumn
Close to the busy produce and flower market at Covent Garden, and amidst the theatre and cafe streets, narrow Endell Street was always extremely busy. On 2 October 1917, many of Endell Street Hospital's staff enjoyed a welcome break to celebrate the wedding of Dr Rachel Champion to Lieutenant Colonel (Dr) Charles Gordon Shaw. Rachel had moved into a room at 25 Wimpole

Street, the home of Dr Octavia Lewin, next door to her Melbourne colleague Dr Vera Scantlebury some weeks before the wedding. Charles was stationed at the No. 1 Australian Auxiliary Hospital at Harefield in Middlesex more than 30 kilometres from London, and he and Rachel were to move into married quarters after their wedding. Dr Lewin provided an afternoon tea in her dining room; the wedding cake was decorated with fresh white heather rather than the traditional icing, as sugar was strictly rationed.

Vera had spent the morning of the wedding day 'sending some poor unfortunates into the land of oblivion with the aid of a bottle of chloroform'.[61] Endell Street's OCs were sad to lose Rachel as she was a good surgeon with almost two years of experience but made light of it by saying that they hoped marriage was not contagious. Stalwart of the Australian expatriate community, Melbourne woman Mary Bage was on hand to give the bride away. A few days later the groom returned to his unit, the 1st Australian Casualty Clearing Station at Bailleul, 90 kilometres west of Boulogne, for the rapid evacuation of the wounded to England.

Part 5

1918

Chapter 6

'The very uselessness and waste of it all'

These wounds do make one feel ill from the very
uselessness and waste of it all besides the agony
and the suffering. [1]

Dr Vera Scantlebury, London, 26 April 1918

As the final year of the Great War began, a new enemy appeared across the battlefields and hospitals of Europe and Britain. An influenza pandemic that began in the spring of 1918 and continued to spread worldwide into 1919 caused the deaths of more people than any other outbreak of infection in history.[2] Influenza appeared first in France and although the first wave of the disease caused widespread illness in soldiers and civilians there were few deaths. However, a second wave came in autumn of 1918 and spread far more rapidly. The mortality rate amongst its victims was much higher than earlier.[3]

By 1918, the Australian women doctors were scattered across Britain and the battlefields of Europe. Four had completed their service and returned to Australia: Lilian Cooper to Brisbane,

Laura Fowler Hope to Adelaide, Helen Sexton to Melbourne and Lucy Gullett to Sydney. Laura Forster lay in a grave in Zaleschiki, a little village in south-east Galicia.

On the Eastern Front, Mary De Garis worked on in her tent as CMO at the SWH field hospital, 140 kilometres north-west of Salonica. More than 100 kilometres to the south of Mary, Elsie Dalyell was bent over her microscope at her laboratory in the bleak hills behind Salonica.

In France, Phoebe Chapple was travelling between the WAAC camps at Abbeville, Étaples and Rouen; the last being where Sydney doctor Marjory Little had begun work in one of the hospital laboratories. Five hundred kilometres to the south, Isabel Ormiston was at work in the historic Limoges' ceramic factory, temporarily converted to a military hospital.

Elizabeth Hamilton-Browne and Katie Ardill would soon arrive in Egypt where Agnes Bennett and Lucy Gullett had served two years before.

Agnes had returned to London after an eventful journey from Sydney via the Panama Canal. Eleanor Bourne was up in the north of England as Area Controller of the Northern Command of the WAAC at York, and Irene Eaton was in charge of the Eastern Command. In London, Grace Cordingley was beginning her third year at the Royal Free Hospital in Holborn, barely half a kilometre from the Endell Street Military Hospital where Vera Scantlebury was in the operating theatre daily. Emma Buckley was at work in her laboratory at the King George in central London, and all three were experiencing the rush that accompanied the German Spring Offensive. Their last months of war service were filled with work, anxiety, fear and hope.

Glasgow, Scotland

April 1918, Spring

Dr Agnes Bennett had recovered from the serious attack of malaria that caused her return to the Bennett family home in Sydney, and by early 1918 was back in Wellington, New Zealand, where she had developed a large medical practice before the war. By March she was feeling fit and wanted to serve again; to 'get back into the war'.[4] It was difficult to get a berth but she joined the cargo ship *Essex*, again as MO, which was sailing to England via the newly opened Panama Canal, a much longer route than the usual trip through the Suez.

The trip was an alarming experience. The *Essex* called in at Kingston, Jamaica, to collect an anti-submarine gun and the gunner crew, and then sailed north to Halifax in Nova Scotia, Canada, to join a convoy of twenty-three ships to cross the North Atlantic. Halifax was a devastating sight. On 6 December 1917, a French ship carrying a cargo of explosives had collided with a Norwegian freighter and the massive explosion had laid waste to a large part of the town and killed 2000 people. As the *Essex* crossed to England, German U-boats constantly threatened the convoy and thick fog required vigilant manoeuvring. Agnes' boat was involved in one collision and a continual blizzard added to the general anxiety.

The *Essex* reached London safely and the SWH asked Agnes to visit their headquarters in Edinburgh to recount her experiences as CMO of her unit in Ostrovo. While there, she heard that the Glasgow Royal Infirmary was crowded with general and military patients and desperately needed a medical officer. She immediately responded. The staffing situation was dire: the hospital, which normally had fifteen to twenty resident doctors, now had only Agnes and one other doctor. With more than a thousand beds, Agnes found the work extremely taxing, particularly when, after two months, in around mid-1918, the influenza pandemic reached the Scottish cities. Over half the nursing staff went down with the illness and the other doctor died. Agnes had to use second- and third-year medical students to assist in the operating theatre and to give anaesthetics. The operations were often on female munitions workers from local factories, where accidents were commonplace.

By late October, Agnes was completely exhausted and had to resign from the position. She headed first to Edinburgh for two days of uninterrupted sleep and then towards London.

London, England

The WAAC, 1917–1919

In contrast to its name, the British Women's Army Auxiliary Corps or the WAAC, was hardly an 'auxiliary' organisation. In 1917 and 1918 more than 57,000 women served with the organisation and, in 1918, it despatched women doctors to France with responsibility for the health of WAAC members on the Western Front.

In 1914 Dr Letitia Fairfield had been 'longing to get to the Front' but had been told that the war could be won without women doctors when she tried to enlist shortly after its beginning.[5] Letitia had won a Carnegie Scholarship to study medicine at the Edinburgh College of Medicine for Women in 1901 and in 1917 she was appointed as a medical officer for the WAAC, quickly becoming Area Medical Controller of their Southern Command with responsibility for the recruitment and management of many women doctors.[6]

The RAMC had nine command areas. Six of these – Northern, Southern, Eastern, Western, Aldershot and London District – most likely had WAAC Medical Controllers; while the other three – Scottish, Irish and Jersey Commands – probably did not. Six Australian women doctors worked for the WAAC or – its later name – the QMAAC, between 1917 and 1919. Eleanor Bourne, Letitia Fairfield and Irene Eaton were medical controllers for the Northern, Southern and Eastern Commands respectively, and Hilda Esson, Phoebe Chapple and Rachel Champion were medical officers.

Eleanor Bourne had been serving for nineteen months at the Endell Street Military Hospital when she joined the WAAC at Christmas time in 1917. Her colleague Dr Vera Scantlebury missed her friend terribly because she was excellent company, with a great sense of humour, and helped to keep everyone's spirits up. They had celebrated Eleanor's thirty-ninth birthday in early December with dinner at Maison Lyon in Shaftesbury Avenue in London and on Christmas Eve the two WAAC wards at Endell Street Hospital had won the prizes awarded by the OCs for the best Christmas decorations. Eleanor wrote:

> For weeks beforehand a choir had been practising Christmas carols and, early on Christmas morning, carrying lanterns to light them through the blackout, clad in sheets and crowned with holly, the singing procession passed through the wards announcing the great day had come.[7]

Eleanor was posted to York as the Medical Controller of the Northern Command and promoted to the honorary rank of Major, but without any of the entitlements regarding taxation and travel benefits that applied to male officers. She wrote to Vera in February 1918 to say that she was happy in her work with the WAAC but was feeling rather lonely without the tight-knit Endell Street community.

Irene Eaton had been amongst the first group of women doctors to arrive on Malta in 1916 and she had completed her year's contract with the RAMC there in October 1917. Immediately on her return to England, she was posted to the WAAC as Area Medical Controller of the Eastern Command and started work on 17 October. Irene had completed a Diploma of Public Health and had also worked as a pathologist and was well qualified to educate the Eastern Command's doctors in supervision of camps, sanitation and kitchens.

Dr Hilda Bull Esson was a University of Melbourne colleague of Rachel Champion and Vera Scantlebury and had arrived in London from America with her journalist and playwright husband Louis Buvelot Esson in late 1917. The Essons moved into a small flat and soon became part of the Melbourne expatriate social group. Hilda's income as a doctor was the couple's bread and butter and she was immediately employed by the WAAC on a travelling medical board. In February 1918 she was in the northern city of York and her work involved examining women recruits for the various departments of the WAAC. She remained in that role until her pregnancy precluded it and her son Hugh was born in London on 1 May 1918.[8]

Another married member of the WAAC was Hilda's Melbourne University colleague Rachel Champion, who had resigned from her position at the Endell Street Military Hospital after her marriage in October 1917. Rachel still wished to contribute to the war effort and her new husband, Charles, had been posted to France. She worked for the WAAC in London at times during late 1917 and the first months of 1918.

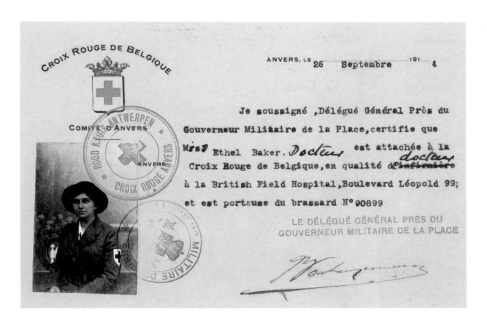

Dr Ethel Baker's Belgian Red Cross accreditation, 1915. *(Dr RCF Stephens)*

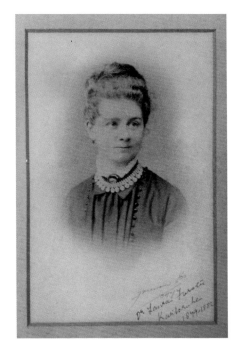

Dr Laura Forster *(Rob L Wagner & Women's College, University of Sydney)*

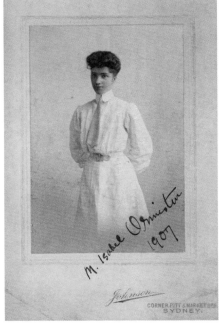

Dr Isabel Ormiston *(NSW State Archives & Records)*

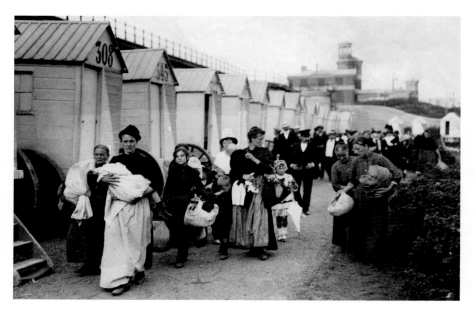

Ostend, Belgium, October 1914: Belgian refugee families leaving their temporary shelters – bathing boxes along the beachfront – to board boats to England. *(Alamy)*

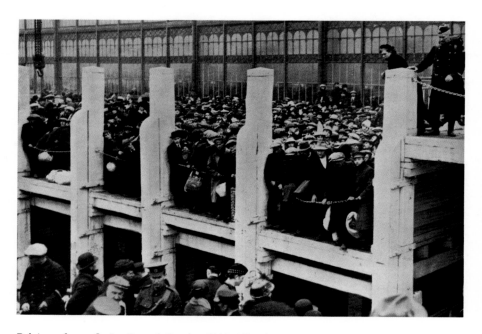

Belgian refugees fleeing Ostend, October 1914. *(Alamy)*

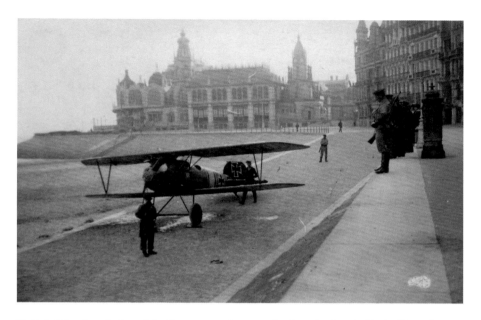

Dr Isabel Ormiston's view of the German army's occupation from her hospital in Le Kursaal, Ostend, Belgium, October 1914. *(Art.com)*

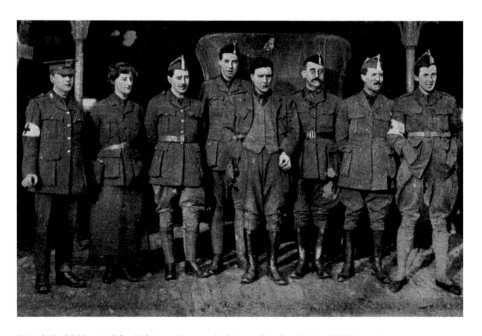

British Field Hospital for Belgium, Furnes, Belgium, October 1914. *(HS Souttar)*

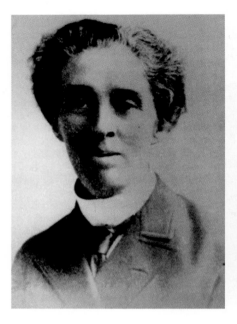

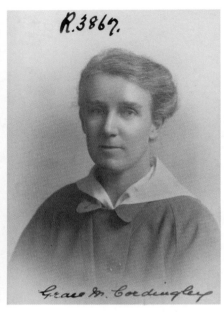

Dr Lilian Cooper *(State Library of Queensland)*

Dr Grace Cordingley *(NSW State Archives & Records)*

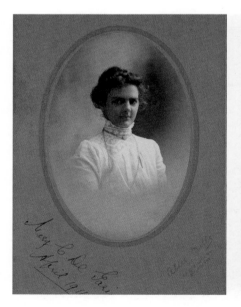

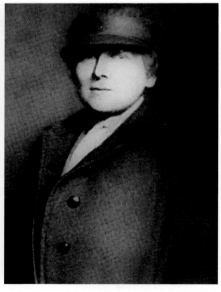

Dr Mary De Garis *(NSW State Archives & Records)*

Dr Elsie Dalyell in RAMC uniform *(University of Sydney Archives)*

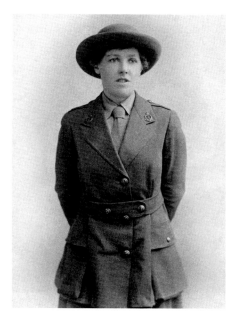

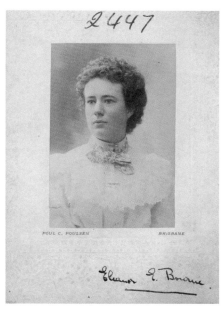

Dr Letitia Fairfield *(Royal Hardie, Salisbury)*

Dr Eleanor Bourne *(NSW State Archives & Records)*

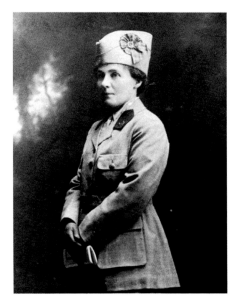

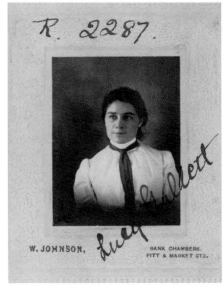

Dr Laura Fowler Hope in the uniform of the Scottish Women's Hospital, c. August 1915. *(State Library of South Australia)*

Dr Lucy Gullett *(NSW State Archives & Records)*

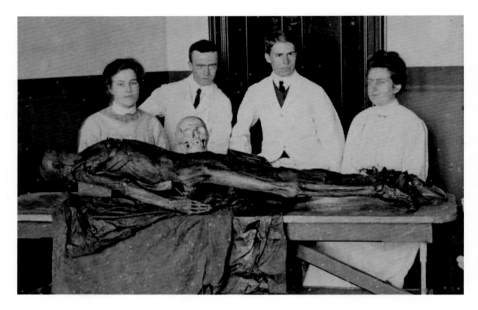

Dr Elizabeth Hamilton-Browne, far right, one of the first two women prosectors appointed by the University of Sydney's Faculty of Medicine, 1906. *(University of Sydney Medical School Online Museum & Archive)*

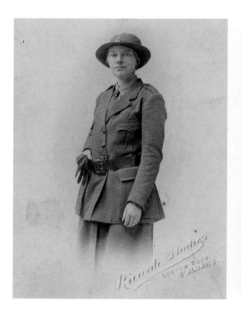

Dr Katie Ardill *(William Girling)*

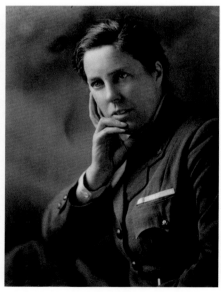

Dr Agnes Bennett in the uniform of the Scottish Women's Hospital, c. August 1916. *(Imperial War Museum, UK)*

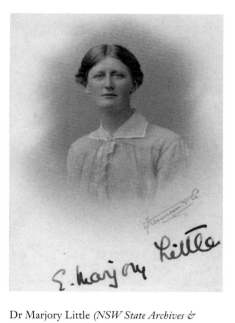

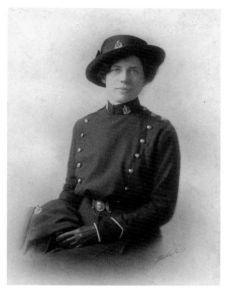

Dr Marjory Little *(NSW State Archives & Records)*

Dr Phoebe Chapple in the uniform of the WAAC/QMAAC *(Australian War Memorial P10871.005)*

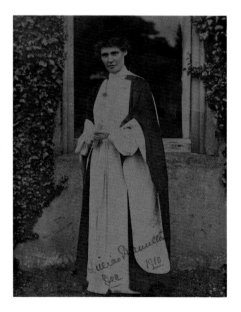

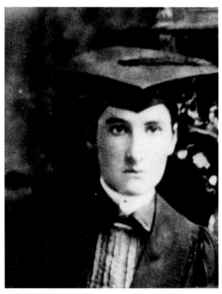

Dr Lillias Hamilton *(Museum of English Rural Life, University of Reading)*

Dr Helen Sexton *(University of Melbourne Archives)*

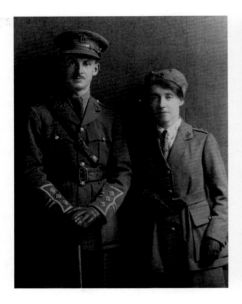

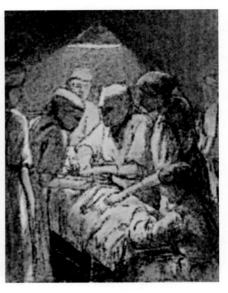

Dr Vera Scantlebury in the uniform of the Women's Hospital Corps with her brother, Dr Cliff Scantlebury, AAMC, July 1918. *(Catherine James Bassett & University of Melbourne Archives)*

'An operation at the Endell Street Military Hospital, London, 1917', by Francis Dodd. *(Wellcome Institute for the History of Medicine, UK)*

Below: Staff of the Endell Street Military Hospital, London, August 1916. Dr Elizabeth Hamilton-Browne is seated 13th from the left, with Dr Rachel Champion immediately to her left. *(The Women's Library, London School of Economics)*

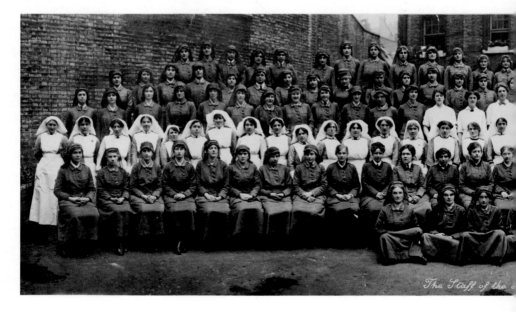

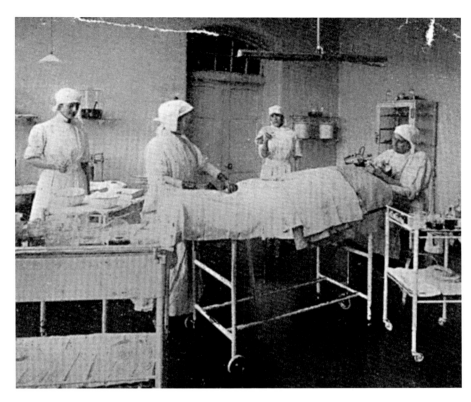

Operating theatre at the Endell Street Military Hospital, London. *(Wellcome Institute for the History of Medicine, UK)*

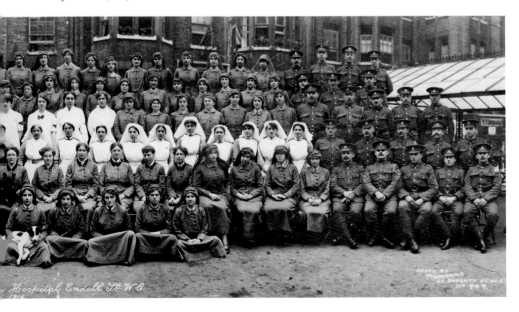

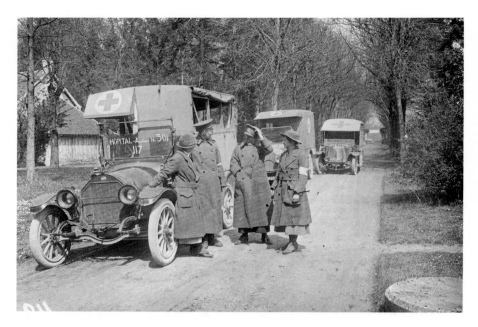

VAD ambulance drivers waiting to pick up the wounded outside the SWH at Abbaye de Royaumont, Asnières-sur-Oise, France, 1915. *(Australian War Memorial P01352.004)*

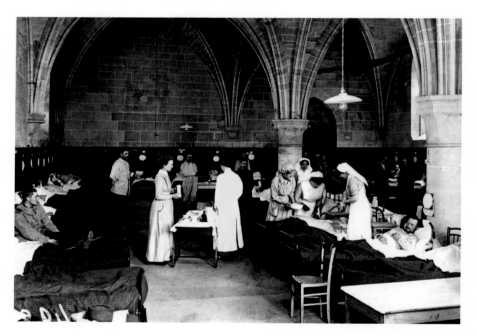

SWH ward set up in the refectory of the Abbaye de Royaumont, Asnières-sur-Oise, France. *(Jacques Moreau/Bridgeman images)*

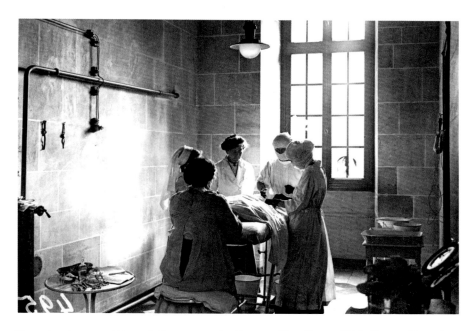

Operating theatre at Abbaye de Royaumont, Asnières-sur-Oise, France, 1915. *(Jacques Moreau/ Bridgeman images)*

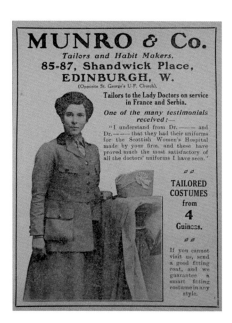

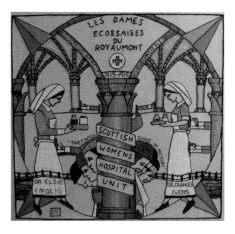

Tailoring advertisement for women doctors in *The Common Cause*, suffrage news journal, 27 August 1915. *(Dr Jennian Geddes)*

'They Will Shine in History', Scottish Diaspora Tapestry panel celebrating the SWH unit at Abbaye de Royaumont, Asnières-sur-Oise, France, stitched by Andrea Cooley. *(Prestoungrange Arts Festival)*

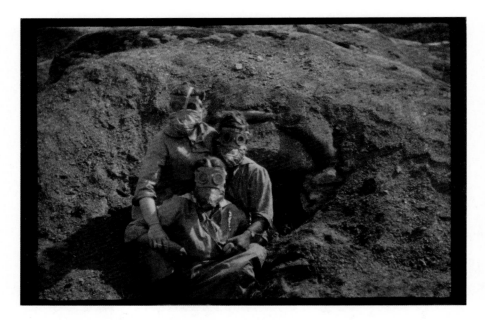

SWH orderlies in gas masks at the entrance to a dugout at a forward dressing station, Dobraveni, c. 1917. *(Alexander Turnbull Library Collection, National Library of New Zealand)*

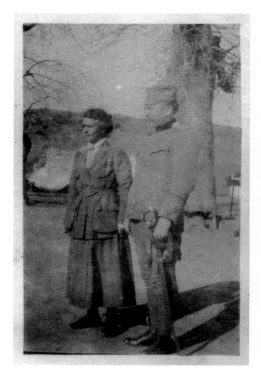

Dr Mary De Garis with a colonel of the Serbian Army, Ostrovo, c. 1917. *(Mitchell Library, Glasgow)*

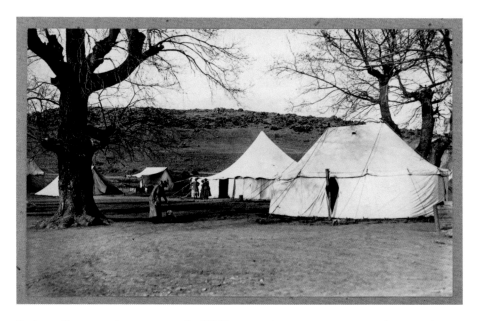

Dr Agnes Bennett at the entrance to the SWH camp at Ostrovo, c. 1917. (*Alexander Turnbull Library Collection, National Library of New Zealand*)

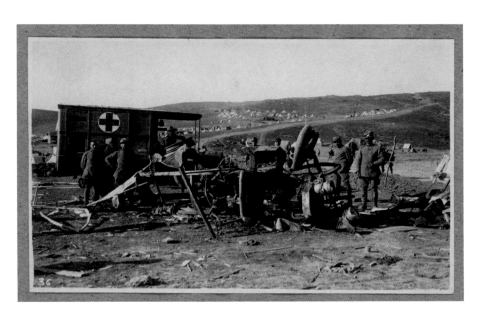

SWH ambulance destroyed by an air raid, camp in the background. (*Alexander Turnbull Library Collection, National Library of New Zealand*)

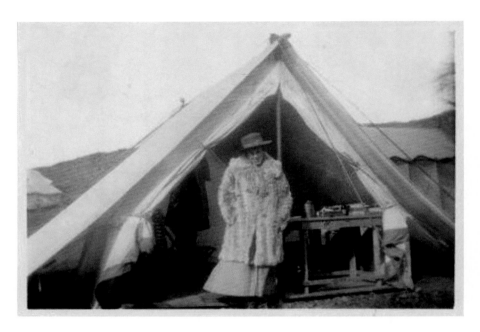

Dr Agnes Bennett outside her tent, Ostrovo, winter 1916–17. *(Alexander Turnbull Library Collection, National Library of New Zealand)*

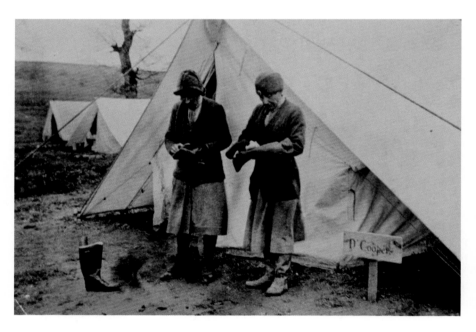

Dr Lilian Cooper, right, wearing SWH hat, and Josephine Bedford, who maintained the SWH ambulance fleet. *(Alexander Turnbull Library Collection, National Library of New Zealand)*

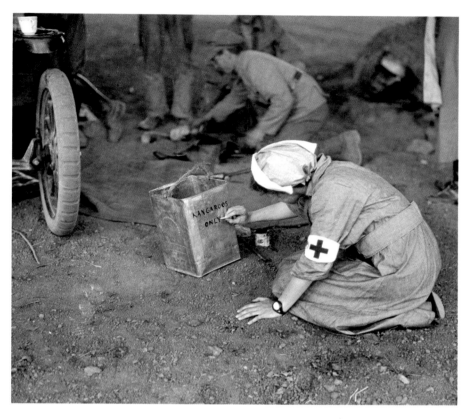

An Australian orderly painting 'Kangaroos Only' on a water can, SWH camp, Ostrovo, 1916. *(Imperial War Museum, UK)*

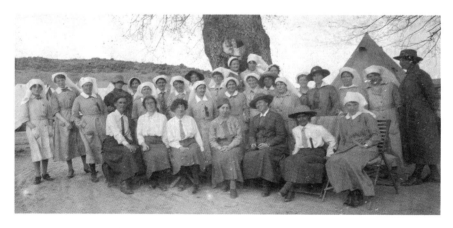

SWH unit at Ostrovo, 1917. Dr Mary De Garis is seated second from right, Dr Agnes Bennett seated third from right and orderly Stella Miles Franklin standing far left. *(Mitchell Library, Glasgow)*

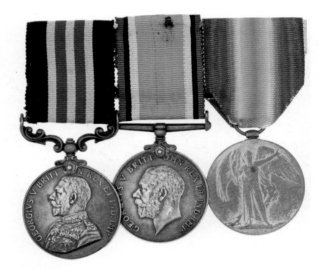

Right: Dr Phoebe Chapple's
WWI medals. From left:
Military Medal, British
War Medal, Victory Medal.
*(Australian War Memorial
REL02991.002)*

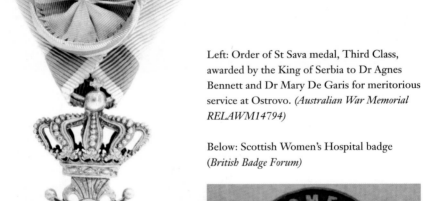

Left: Order of St Sava medal, Third Class,
awarded by the King of Serbia to Dr Agnes
Bennett and Dr Mary De Garis for meritorious
service at Ostrovo. *(Australian War Memorial
RELAWM14794)*

Below: Scottish Women's Hospital badge
(British Badge Forum)

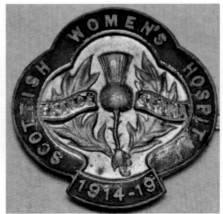

Western Front: Abbeville, France

November 1917, Autumn

Over in France, Dr Phoebe Chapple arrived in Abbeville in November 1917 as one of the first two women doctors working for the WAAC in an overseas posting. Abbeville, on the river Somme, was the headquarters for all lines of Allied communication during the war and home to the 3rd Australian General Hospital as well as the South African and British military hospitals. The town was 45 kilometres west of Amiens, and was a crucial train and road junction; taking Amiens was a major objective of the German army's Spring Offensive. Abbeville, with its vital role in communications, was very vulnerable to aerial bombardment throughout April, May and June of 1918. After the war, the town would be awarded the French Croix de Guerre medal for its faithful contribution to the war effort while under constant bombardment from the German air force.

Phoebe was wearing her new light grey WAAC uniform with RAMC badges in place but without any badges or insignia of rank. The uniform was clearly that of an officer and easily distinguished from the WAAC's 'workers' ubiquitous khaki jacket and skirt, which had to be no more than 12 inches (30 centimetres) from the ground. Wearing the RAMC badges was entirely at the discretion of the local CO and some directed women doctors to remove them.

Phoebe was unperturbed by her proximity to the battle front, even fatalistic, because there was so much work to do.

> You just felt you were in God's hands, and if you were killed while fulfilling the duty of the moment, then it could not be helped; and it was no more than those wonderful soldiers were doing incessantly.[9]

She travelled between the WAAC camps at Étaples, Abbeville and Rouen, 150 kilometres apart, and later to Le Havre, to examine sick and injured corps women. She also inspected the sanitary conditions in the women's camps, billets and work places. Anyone who required hospitalisation could be sent to the two WAAC wards at the Endell Street Military Hospital back in London. This was where Dr Vera Scantlebury discovered one of her fellow lodgers, Miss Rundle, who had been working as a driver with the WAAC in France, in February 1918.

Abbeville and Étaples, with their important communications and administrative centres and major hospitals, were targets for German bombers, and a series of raids on the bases in the Somme began in late March.[10] In mid-May 1918, the people of Abbeville and its camps and hospitals observed the familiar drift of white leaflets floating down from enemy planes. The missives warned of impending bombing and some townspeople took to sleeping in the open countryside.

Tuesday 21 May was cloudless with a full moon. At 11 pm the WAAC camp attached to the army's No. 2 Army Supply Depot was awakened by the rapid fire of anti-aircraft guns and machine guns. Everyone dashed for the slit trenches near their huts and tents where they remained for five hours until an aerial torpedo, looking like a ball of fire turning over and over, hit the camp. One woman had to be dug out and another evacuated to hospital in England. Only four of the camp's seventeen huts survived.[11]

Eight days later, on 29 May, Phoebe was attending the camp and, as the only doctor on duty, was asked to stay for the night. At 4 am the planes returned and the bombardment was deafening. Bombs set alight a lorry close to the WAAC camp and, by its light, three more bombs were dropped. Two of them hit empty huts vacated by the women but a third struck part of a covered zigzag trench where forty women were sheltering. Nine WAAC members were killed and another seven wounded. Alice Thomasson, Mary Blaikley, Beatrice Campbell and Catherine Connor died instantly and Jennie Watson a short time later. The five women were all corps members who undertook general domestic work. Also killed were Jennie McKerral, who was a postal clerk; Annie Moores, a cook; and dining room staff Ethel Parker and Margaret Caswell.[12]

Along with the unit's administrator, Mrs Gibson, clerk Ethel Cartlege and Sophie Cross from camp administration, Phoebe left the cover of the trench immediately to give whatever first aid and comfort she could. She worked frantically with limited medical supplies, tending to the dead and wounded as bombs continued to fall around them. Sophie had been knocked down by the initial explosion but scrambled up to help Phoebe with the injured. Ethel, whose shoes had been blown off by the explosion, hurried from one wounded woman to another, reassuring and comforting them despite a nail embedded in her foot.

Other women showed similar courage and resolve that night. QMAAC Sister Jane Trotter was in charge in the nearby hospital wards when the raid began. The orderly working beside her was killed in the first explosion but Sister Trotter continued to calmly work her way through the wards, checking on the condition of her patients. A fellow nurse, Ethel Watkins, stayed to help her patients despite being injured by shrapnel; and another, Agnes Parker, worked on in her ward when it was badly damaged by a bomb early in the raid. Mary Stubbs, a member of the First Aid Nursing Yeomanry (FANY), was given the role of evacuating the wounded and was waiting in the driver's seat of her car as two wounded were loaded. A bomb landed 30 metres away and the stretcher-bearers ran for a trench but Mary refused to go with them and stayed in the car to reassure her passengers.

All eight women earned a Military Cross that night but, as
none held a commission – not even Phoebe with the honorary
rank of major – they each received a Military Medal instead. A
special supplement of the *London Gazette* in October 1918 noted
that the medals were awarded for 'gallantry and devotion to duty
during an air-raid'.[13] Phoebe did not look at her work that way. She
wrote, 'I think when there is suffering and death near at hand, fear
absents itself.'[14]

After the raid, communications were down for some time but
eventually field ambulances arrived to take the wounded women
given emergency treatment by Phoebe to the local military hospitals. Sophie Cross called the roll as groups of women huddled
together clad in their pyjamas and blankets. Tears fell quietly
when there was no reply to a name.

Two days later their dead colleagues were buried with full
military honours. The coffins were taken by gun carriages to the
cemetery and the Royal Air Force flew overhead. In one coffin was
Alice Thomasson, a 21-year-old cotton mill worker from Bolton
in north-west England, who had signed up for domestic work and
been in the camp for only three days when the bomb struck. Six
months later the WO sent a parcel to her family containing some
of her belongings, including a nightdress, a photo locket, a piece
of shrapnel, a haversack, scissors and pencils.

Alongside Alice in the trench was fellow domestic worker
Beatrice Campbell, who had previously worked for eighteen
months in the 'Devil's Porridge' Munitions Factory in Gretna,
Scotland, producing cordite shells. Beatrice was twenty and her
headstone in the Abbeville Cemetery reads 'In remembrance of
dear Beatrice, beloved of all who knew her'. The nine WAAC
women who died together in the trench lie side by side in Section
238C of the cemetery.

Western Front: Rouen and Étaples, France

April 1918, Spring

In the laboratory of the 25th Stationary Hospital in Rouen, Sydney doctor Marjory Little had begun working with Dr Charles Martin from London's Lister Institute. The Lister was known as the 'Central Laboratory' throughout the war and Martin was well acquainted with Australian pathologists. He had employed Dr Emma Buckley, a University of Sydney and Women's College colleague of Marjory, earlier in the war years.

Eight of the Sydney women doctors who went to war were associated through the Women's College, which would remain an important part of Marjory's life. Marjory had degrees in both science and medicine but it was histopathology, the changes in human tissue caused by disease, which really interested her. Histopathology requires finely detailed work examining biological tissues under a microscope.

Marjory had wanted to serve since her graduation in 1915 but instead had been at Sydney's Royal Prince Alfred Hospital, replacing the Chief Pathologist, Dr Arthur Tebbutt, while he was overseas with the AIF. Tebbutt returned to Sydney late in 1917 and Dr Elsie Dalyell had written from her laboratory at the No. 63 Hospital north of Salonica to tell Marjory that the RAMC were looking for pathologists, particularly bacteriologists.[15] In 1918, it was difficult to obtain a passage on board one of the ships that were crammed with military personnel and to acquire official permission to travel to England. But after several months of persisting, Marjory eventually reached England in late March 1918.

Marjory went straight to the Lister Institute on the Chelsea Embankment in London. The institute's appearance – it looked a little like a wedding cake in 1918 – belied the gravity of the work taking place inside: the pursuit of the bacteria that caused so many deaths during the Great War. She was greeted by English microbiologist Dr Harriette Chick, who was involved in the diagnosis of typhoid and other common diseases in the trenches. She told Marjory that Sir (Dr) Charles Martin was in urgent need of a bacteriologist in his laboratory at Rouen over in France.

When Marjory approached the WO, however, they seemed uncertain about employing her and about whether they could find her accommodation. A few days later an envelope arrived at her flat. It was delivered by a King's Messenger wearing his embossed gold badge with a tiny silver greyhound hanging from the base – the tradition of royal messengers had existed since the fifteenth century. Marjory sat looking at the letter, marked 'Secret' in thick black letters, for several minutes before opening it. It contained an order to report to Dr Martin at the 25th British Stationary Hospital in Rouen; she had been given the nominal rank of captain with the RAMC.[16]

The ancient city of Rouen, on the river Seine, was a major logistics centre for the Allies during the war. It was one of the main British Infantry Base Depots, receiving men on arrival from England and training them until they were posted to a unit at the front. It was also a supply depot and home to ten British hospitals and the No. 1 Australian General Hospital.

When Marjory was posted to Rouen in early April 1918, Dr Martin was also Director of the British Expeditionary Force laboratories in Paris and Trouville. On arrival at the 25th Hospital Marjory found that Martin, the entire laboratory staff, several nurses and twenty-six orderlies were ill with high fevers, which appeared to be the Spanish influenza that the newspapers had recently been describing.

Dr Sydney Patterson, who would become the first Director of the Walter and Eliza Hall Institute of Research in Pathology in Melbourne in late 1919, was in charge of a nearby hospital that had sent several patients to the 25th.[17] His unit had received a hospital-trainload of patients mostly with malaria and sandfly fever, but many had also suffered from a highly contagious three- to five-day fever during the journey, as had the accompanying RAMC personnel. Some of the patients had died and Marjory began immediately on the bacteriological analysis of the samples taken at autopsies.[18]

Marjory worked with Eleanor Williams, a talented nurse who was from the Adelaide Hospital and was highly skilled in laboratory procedures. Marjory greatly valued Eleanor's work and congenial personality and said their relationship was a 'perfect laboratory association'.[19] Together they examined the pathology of streptococci and staphylococci, keeping precise records of valuable data. Strep and staph infections caused problems such as blood poisoning, pneumonia and skin abscesses, and strep infections were the main complication of influenza during the war.

Pathology work during the war years revealed quite unexpected results at times. Lance Corporal Aubrey Cumberbatch of the British West Indies Regiment was from Trinidad in tropical Jamaica and arrived in France in August 1917. Within two months he was admitted to the 22nd General Hospital in Camiers with trench foot. The cold of the ensuing French winter and spring must have been miserable for Aubrey. By the end of April 1918 he had arrived at the 25th, and it is likely that Marjory's tests confirmed that Aubrey was not ill with the influenza that was beginning to dominate their work, but was afflicted with leprosy.

After a month of pathology tests and treatment at the 25th Stationary Hospital he was repatriated to his new home – the

Leper Home in Spanish Town, Jamaica.[20] By the time Aubrey reached home, Marjory and Eleanor were hard at work on the pathology and bacteriology of the influenza bacterium that was indiscriminately hitting the military and civilians on both sides.

After some months, they were posted to Étaples, where Marjory took charge of the 46th Stationary Hospital's laboratory. The 46th was an isolation hospital in the largest army base camp ever established overseas by the British, and contained one of the army's most important laboratories. Although Marjory's new position carried the rank of major, she remained a captain but was given a small salary increase.

The army base at Étaples could house up to 100,000 people, and its hospitals had a capacity of 22,000 patients.[21] The wards were in long wooden huts with tarred canvas roofs and stood in dozens of neat rows connected by cinder paths. Marjory and Eleanor lived in one of the rows of small Alwyn huts – simple wooden-framed structures with canvas walls.

Elsie Tranter, an Australian nurse at the 26th General Hospital, also in Étaples, called the town 'the land of hospitals' and said that they stretched for 6 kilometres.[22] Elsie's hospital was on a slight slope and ran along the railway line which followed the river Canche south from the town. On the other side were sand dunes and the sea, and most days the fishing fleet with its reddish brown sails could be seen going out to sea during the hospital's lunch hour. Elsie wrote about the ghastly wounds and amputations she saw in the operating theatre but also wrote:

> The outside world is still very beautiful – flowers everywhere – mignonette, bluebells and daisies. In peacetime this spot where the camp is, is a favourite artists' resort as the sunrise and sunset effects here are supposed to be the finest in the world.[23]

Marjory's hospital, the 46th, stood at the edge of a dense pine forest that covered thousands of hectares, interrupted only by the narrow poplar-lined roads common in the Picardy region of France. She wrote of the brilliant yellow poplars in autumn and the roving herds of deer but it was spring and summer that she liked best, when the laboratory doors stood wide open.

> Then those to whom the forest had become a close friend knew where to find the glades where the primroses and the lilies-of-the-valley flowered; then the apple trees in the old orchard amongst which nestled the brown huts of the Sister's Mess burst into masses of delicate colour . . . the cold and discomforts of the winter were forgotten.[24]

As mentioned by Elsie Tranter, Étaples was also home to an artists' colony that included Australian artist Iso Rae, who lived beside the river near the camp's southern tip. Iso remained in Étaples throughout the war and her pastel drawings of life in a huge camp behind the lines were completed in snippets of time away from her work as a VAD at one of the YMCA huts.[25]

The 46th Hospital contained nearly 1000 hospital beds, and Marjory's laboratory 'consisted of a long, narrow, working-room with small storeroom and kitchen opening off one end, and beyond these the animal house, where lived our rabbits, guinea-pigs, mice, white rats and occasionally monkeys'.[26]

In the lab, rabbits were used to diagnose diphtheria and guinea pigs to identify tuberculosis. Conditions were primitive – gas was not available in the laboratory so the autoclaves and ovens were heated with huge primus stoves, and Bunsen burners were replaced with spirit lamps. In the coldest months, everything in the laboratory would freeze overnight and Marjory worried about the effect on the cultures stored there. The post-mortem hut had neither heating nor hot water and in winter Marjory's fingers were numb and her feet 'reduced to blocks of ice'.[27]

She was, however, delighted to be working again with the highly trained Eleanor Williams, whom she regarded as an accomplished bacteriologist. And at Christmas time in 1918, everyone enjoyed Eleanor's cake made from sugar and dried fruit, most likely sent from EC De Garis & Co, Mildura, Australia, and baked in the laboratory's oven.

With Eleanor, Marjory worked on every type of infectious disease that presented in patients at the 46th and surrounding hospitals. When the pathologist from the venereal centre at the 51st Hospital in Étaples was absent, they took on that work too. Her OC, Colonel SL Cummins, had been Professor of Pathology at the RAMC College before the war and Adviser in Pathology to the Director General of Medical Services in France. He wrote to Charles Martin that he had a very high opinion of Marjory's excellent detailed work and that he was greatly indebted to her.[28]

Marjory was not hard to like; she was a warm person, genuinely interested in people, and had a great sense of humour. Undoubtedly a strong personality, she was meticulous in everything she attempted and Cummins clearly recognised this quality in her pathology work.[29]

In 1918 there were 2 million soldiers in camps across northern France and they had come from all over the world. The constant movement of people and animals encouraged contagion, and Étaples became an epicentre of the 1918 flu pandemic.

Laboratories across the Western Front and in Britain were working on the aetiology of this particular strain of influenza and Marjory and Eleanor were keen to contribute. Based on fatal influenza cases in Rouen and Étaples, they co-authored a paper on influenza pathology, which Cummins regarded as one of the best, and which was included in a Special Report of the British Medical Research Council into influenza.

Influenza was not the only concern at Étaples. Marjory's hospital was in a strategically important location, adjacent to the Boulogne–Paris railway line and surrounded by extensive camps of the British, Canadian, Australian and New Zealand armies. Every day, the road that ran past her laboratory was full of ambulances, supply trucks and marching troops coming and going, and at night the truck lights continued past the glow of lighted huts and tents.[30]

From May 1918, around the time Marjory and Eleanor first arrived in Étaples, there were extensive and frightening German bombing raids on the base and the town. On 19 May, a beautiful moonlit night, roads around the camp were shining white and the railway lines silver. At 10.30 pm, when most of the camp was asleep, a ferocious attack began and 150 bombs were dropped over two hours from thirty German planes.[31] The death toll was high: 168 patients and a nurse were killed and 622 were wounded, including eleven nurses.

At the 46th Hospital, several patients were killed or wounded, and a nurse was killed during another raid on 1 June. A subsequent attack on 12 August killed two officers but the staff had managed to get all the patients out of the wards and safely into the recently created dugouts. Marjory and Eleanor worked on, regardless of the bombing raids and the newly observed and highly infectious influenza.

Chapter 7

'This wholesale slaughter cannot go on forever'[1]

Dr Vera Scantlebury, London, 1 May 1918

London, England

February 1918, Winter

February 1918 in England and France was fortunately much milder than the dreadfully severe frosts and freezing weather of February 1917. Early in the month, Dr Elizabeth Hamilton-Browne moved into the room that had previously been occupied by Dr Rachel Champion at 25 Wimpole Street in London. After her marriage to Lieutenant Colonel Gordon Shaw, Rachel had moved into the married quarters at the No. 1 Australian Auxiliary Hospital at Harefield outside of London, where her husband was chief surgeon.

Elizabeth's stay was a short one because, after more than two arduous years in the operating theatres of the Endell Street Military Hospital and living through the London bombings, she wanted to move to a different theatre of war. She was readily accepted for work with the RAMC in Egypt with the honorary rank of captain.

In early May she gave a happy farewell lunch for her colleagues at Le Moulin D'Or in central London but Vera Scantlebury was saddened that Elizabeth would soon leave for her service in Egypt. She would miss her company, and the hospital would miss her surgical skill. Vera would be the only Australian remaining at Endell Street, living a 'kaleidoscopic existence'. She observed, 'London where life is seen in so many phases has a strange and powerful fascination drawing people to it though killing them at the same time.'[2]

On 4 May a little group of Endell Street friends waved Elizabeth off at Waterloo Station. She sailed that evening bound for Alexandria and, although the trip across the Mediterranean was still perilous with German submarines patrolling the sea lanes leading to the Suez Canal, she arrived in Egypt safely.

Alexandria/Cairo, Egypt

May 1918, Spring

In January 1915, an Ottoman army led by the Germans had advanced into the Sinai desert to gain control of the Suez Canal. The Sinai was part of the British Protectorate of Egypt and, in response, the Allied Egypt Expeditionary Force (EEF) was created, part of which was the ANZAC Mounted Division. When Elizabeth arrived, the EEF had recently regained the Jordan Rift Valley, where from May to September there was almost no rain and daily temperatures reached 42°C to 46°C. The transportation of water was an enormous problem and dehydration was a formidable foe for both sides.

Elizabeth's posting was to the No. 19 General Hospital in the Hadra district on the eastern side of Alexandria. From

March 1915, the city had been transformed into a massive military camp and hospital centre for British and French troops. Apart from the No. 19, there were the 17th, 21st, 78th and 87th General Hospitals and the No. 5 Indian Hospital. After the Gallipoli campaign ended, Alexandria continued to have an important hospital focus during the subsequent operations in Egypt, the Sinai desert and Palestine.

Elizabeth's hospital was previously a German hospital known as The Deaconesses but it had been rebuilt by the British into a much larger facility. It was an attractive four-storey building with two wings that ended in verandahs decorated with lacework and lattice for sun protection when patients' beds were wheeled outside.[3] The narrow, arched windows were designed to keep out the heat, and the front was later decorated with an intricately carved domed tower.

Alexandria sits on the Mediterranean Sea and its climate is more temperate than Cairo's. Before the war it had been an exotic destination, popular with British, French and German tourists. The shops and street sellers were well stocked when war began and eager to sell to soldiers and medical personnel. Elizabeth wandered the streets where Greek, French and Arab shopkeepers displayed their wares in glass cases out on the footpath, while in their windows were more postcards, antiquities and souvenirs.[4] Street sellers sold roasted corn cobs, flat breads and trinkets and loudly offered shoeshines while women in long dark gowns criss-crossed the streets balancing earthen water jugs on their heads.

Both hospital ships and troopships constantly used Alexandria's seaport and the incessant traffic through the port produced ideal conditions for transporting new epidemics around the globe.

While Elizabeth was involved in tending wounded and sick soldiers of the EEF, who were brought in from the desert battles, her work at the 19th Hospital was much less surgical than at Endell Street Military Hospital. Instead, she was increasingly dealing with men ill with malaria and fevers that had not been encountered before. From June to December 1918 there was

a sudden onset of sickness which far surpassed all calculations. It was a 'blizzard' of malaria and a gust of the world-wind of influenza that caused the sick wave and led to a mortality among friends and foes greater than from the severest battles of the campaign.[5]

The *Magazine of the Women's College* of the University of Sydney noted that Elizabeth also served in Palestine some time in 1918 but unfortunately no other records exist of this posting. Eight women doctors were sent to a 2000-bed hospital on the borders of Palestine to treat surgical and medical cases and infectious diseases and Elizabeth may have been one of them.[6] The hospital was possibly one of those set up in the Deir el Belah–Gaza region near the Palestinian border, established during the first British military offensives of October and November 1917.[7]

Back in southern England, Dr Katie Ardill completed her assignment in Dover in May 1918 and was also posted to Egypt. Cairo was the headquarters of the British garrison in Egypt and Katie's position was at the Citadel Hospital, which had been the garrison's principal pre-war military hospital. The Citadel was her fourth hospital – and Egypt her third country – in three years but it was doubtless the most extraordinary building that Katie had served in. The Citadel is a vast medieval fortress built by Salah-el-Din (Saladin) between 1176 and 1183 as protection from the forces of the Christian Crusade, and it sits on a spur of the Mukattam Hills. Each side of the complex contains a

mosque: the fourteenth-century mosque of Muhammad Ali, and
the Mahmud Pasha mosque built in the sixteenth-century.

The Citadel had been the RAMC headquarters since 1898
and by 1918 its ancient walls were surrounded by army camps.
The No. 19 Hospital was inside the fortress walls and had
beds for 750 patients. The wards where Katie did her morning
rounds were in large pavilions where the summer temperatures
rose consistently to between 40°C and 42°C during the day and
only dropped to 36°C overnight, while it was difficult to heat
them to anything warmer than 13°C in winter. The elevated slit
windows that ran under the ward's lofty ceilings were covered
in mosquito netting, but this still let in the fine sandy dust
which covered the patients, their beds, the floors, everything. It
became especially trying when 'the terrible Khamsin which is
a red-hot hurricane seemingly from the throttle of hades blew
through the wards'.[8]

Katie's patients came from the campaigns in Egypt and the
Sinai Peninsula. At nightfall out in the desert, the wounded were
collected by stretcher-bearers and loaded with great effort onto
camel cacolets, two stretchers with head coverings that ran across
the top of the camel's humps.[9] Or the wounded might be placed in
a sand cart drawn by a mule. These were the only types of transport that could carry the wounded or sick through the fine sand
to the nearest railhead. Getting them to Cairo would often take
all night. In the pale yellows and blues of dawn they would arrive
in convoys, exhausted and in pain but gladdened by the sight of
the Citadel courtyard.

By 1918 Katie was still dealing with surgical cases but just as
many admissions were for illness and the doctors had considerable
difficulty in distinguishing between malignant malaria and influenza.[10] Katie served for fourteen months at the Citadel Hospital

before she was recalled to London in mid-1919, finally returning to Sydney on the SS *Ulysses* in October.

Eastern Front: Ostrovo, Macedonia

June 1918, Summer

Summer had arrived at the Lake Ostrovo field hospital. The beds were full of soldiers suffering mostly with malaria and other fevers and the America Unit's CMO, Mary De Garis, had a large tent erected for the sick women and children who arrived.

In early June, Mary suffered another blow when her mother, Elizabeth, died unexpectedly from a heart attack while staying on Guernsey to recuperate from a bout of pneumonia; possibly Spanish influenza.[11] As for so many people during the war, new grief accrued on older grief, with no time to consider either. The work just continued. Mary felt numb and longed to return to Melbourne to see her father and family. Totally exhausted, she resigned as CMO at the end of September 1918 and made preparations for the long journey home via Rome. Before doing so, Mary took a short break in Switzerland, but instead of resting she insisted on helping the SWH staff who were en route to the Royaumont Hospital in France.

The Ostrovo staff were distressed to see Mary go and wrote her an appreciative letter describing her fairness and how they felt safe under her governance. Mary was a strict disciplinarian, but she also possessed the happy knack of having staff who obeyed and respected her orders while also loving her. They appreciated their 'Chief's' great sense of justice and that she judged each of them on their merits; she was their 'guide, philosopher and friend'.[12] Mary wrote later:

All of the sisters were kind and conscientious workers, and most were among the most capable nurses I have ever met. Without doubt there was an art in living and working in tents, and some acquired it easily and some with difficulty. We are a happy family, in spite of occasional bickerings. There must be few of us who cannot look back on their term of service with the SWH and the Serbs as one of the happiest and most useful periods of their lives.[13]

Former CMO Agnes Bennett agreed: 'Altogether we have had experiences by the score that will remain vivid memories all our lives.'[14]

Mary was anxious to get home to Australia and her family but her departure was delayed. In October 1918, en route to Rome by train, exhaustion and grief finally caught up with her. She fell desperately ill with suspected Spanish influenza, although she described it as 'double pneumonia'. She was discovered in a hotel room, alone and extremely unwell, by some RAMC medical officers who promptly transferred her to the American Red Cross Hospital. Her recovery took six long weeks. The SWH sent Dr Ruth Conway out to Italy to accompany Mary on the trip back to London.

Once she was feeling strong enough, Mary caught a train to Edinburgh to be reunited with the SWH women administrators who had supported her so well during her time as CMO in Ostrovo. They presented Mary with a gold watch and later, in 1919, they gave her a copy of *A History of the Scottish Women's Hospitals* by Eva Shaw McLaren, sister of the SWH founder Dr Elsie Inglis. Mary's letter of thanks praised all of the SWH women: 'I shall always remember my association with the SWH with pleasure. Practical experience has convinced me that women run things very well, making me a more ardent feminist than ever.'[15]

The Serbian government also recognised Mary's war service, decorating her with the Medal of St Sava, 3rd Class, in September 1918, a high honour.[16] She was also awarded the British War Medal and the Victory Medal by the British government but received nothing from the Australian government.

Arriving in Melbourne on the SS *Miltiades* in February 1919, Mary was mentioned in the newspapers as

> more than a simple woman doctor . . . She is a woman war-doctor who spent her time in the Big Upheaval driving her car through Serbia succouring and healing [with an] interesting collection of souvenirs and curios, many made from shells and cartridges and some from a German zeppelin.[17]

Reunited with her father, siblings, nephews and nieces at their home in the Melbourne suburb of Sandringham, she was looking for a medical position away from the city. It appears that she may have had contacts in Geelong because by May, she was proudly driving her car to Geelong to establish a private practice in Victoria's second largest city.

London, England

June 1918, Summer
As a result of the 1918 German Spring Offensive, hospitals in London during May and June were busy and the wards at the Endell Street Military Hospital constantly full. Endell Street's OCs asked Dr Vera Scantlebury to call in on some young Australian soldiers in one of the wards.

A young South Australian asked me 'Do you come from Australia? Go on! It's nice to see an Australian girl again. And you came over all by yourself? That was plucky' and so on. Much later when I had gone he found out much to his embarrassment that I was one of the doctors.[18]

Vera was about to sign on for another six months and wondered if the war would ever end. Londoners now had ration cards for meats, bacon, fat, sugar and coal, and little shrines to fallen soldiers were appearing on many of London's streets.

Dr Letitia Fairfield was still working in London, serving as Area Controller for the WAAC's Southern Command. But in June 1918 she was recruited as CMO for the newly formed Women's Royal Air Force (WRAF).[19]

Until 1918, Britain's newly developing air force consisted of two sections: the Royal Flying Corps was part of the British army, while the British navy controlled the Royal Naval Air Force. In April, the two were merged to form the Royal Air Force (RAF), which led to the formation of the WRAF as an auxiliary organisation of the RAF. Like the army and the WAAC, women's involvement in the air force was intended to replace and therby free up men for active service and thousands of women wanted to join up. Brit Helen Gwynne-Vaughan, previously Chief Controller of the WAAC, was appointed as WRAF Commandant and designed the new blue uniforms with their badge dominated by a white bird and the motto *Per Arduo ad Astra* – Through Struggle to the Stars.

As the WRAF's CMO, Letitia had responsibility for the medical care of 8000 personnel who lived in military quarters and another 22,000 who lived at home. It was intended that she have twelve to fourteen women doctors in her team, but even women doctors were now in short supply and she could not recruit more than four or five. Her colleagues found her to be delightful and vigorous, but in coping with such a demanding role Letitia could also be dogmatic and at times infuriating.[20]

Letitia was honoured to serve and she was delighted to fly between air force bases with her male colleagues.[21] Women, however, were not permitted to board an aeroplane in Britain during the war and Letitia had to obtain special permission from the RAF's Commandant, Richard Munday, whose sorties in his Sopwith Camel were legendary.[22] She fumed over the inequalities regarding the status of women doctors that continued until the end of the war, writing that the conditions of service for medical women were deplorable and only accepted on the grounds of grave national emergency.

Like many of the women doctors who served during the war, Letitia was given an honorary rank only, as a lieutenant colonel, but her uniform was unadorned with any evidence of rank, although she was permitted to wear RAMC badges on her lapels. She liked to write about the reaction of the military when they first met her on arrival at a camp, saying that she never knew

> whether one is going to be received as a sort of head cook by a junior subaltern (very rarely) or . . . treated as a member of the Higher Command and find the Colonel and the next six officers in the camp waiting . . . in the latter instance the Adjutant gave the show away by bursting into giggles and saying to the Colonel, 'We didn't expect a lady, did we, sir?'.[23]

Letitia worked with the WRAF from mid-1918 until well into 1920, when the women's air force was finally disbanded. She did not receive the fully commissioned rank of lieutenant colonel until the WO sought her expertise in 1940, when another grave emergency beckoned. During that conflict, she was appointed as the Senior Women's Medical Officer of the Armed Forces.

Edinburgh, Scotland

1918, Summer

When Dr Mabel Murray-Prior arrived in Edinburgh in mid-1918, the Edinburgh War Hospital, Scotland's largest military hospital, was crammed to overflowing with more than 3000 patients. The environment was in sharp contrast to Mabel's previous appointment at Royal Herbert Military Hospital in Greenwich, where the building was of grand proportions.

Until 1915, the Edinburgh War Hospital had been the Bangour Village Hospital, a psychiatric facility based on a village plan with individual two-storey villas on a farm, including 80 hectares of woodlands. The hospital had its own railway line linked to the Uphall Station 3 kilometres away, and Mabel would have arrived at the hospital station as many of the staff did, daily.[24] As the hospital's villas filled with patients, additional marquees were erected and pre-fabricated huts appeared around the extensive grounds. Much of Mabel's work was with recuperating soldiers, but sometimes secondary operations were necessary to improve the rate of healing. Wounded and sick soldiers, many with influenza, continued to arrive and Mabel remained at work at the EWH for several months into 1919.

While Mabel endured the Scottish winter, Elsie Dalyell remained at Salonica with the 63rd General Hospital, where the winter temperature hovered around a more comfortable 10°C to 11°C.

At the end of the war, the 82nd General Hospital was sent from Salonica to Constantinople to help with the outbreak of a cholera epidemic. Having developed considerable expertise in the diagnosis of cholera and a range of enteric fevers, Elsie was sent to the Turkish capital as bacteriologist for the 82nd in early 1919. Refugees had swollen the city's population to a million and over-crowding, malnutrition and poor sanitation combined to create a perfect storm for the outbreak of fevers such as cholera.

Elsie remained in Turkey until July 1919 and was awarded an OBE in June that year as well as being 'Mentioned in Dispatches' in both 1918 and 1919 for outstanding service. She served for four and a half years in six different countries – Serbia, England, France, Malta, Greece and Turkey – and saved countless lives with her untiring efforts in providing the correct diagnoses.

The influenza pandemic in 1918 and 1919 meant that the demand for medical services remained strong. Eveline Cohen had completed her twelve-month contract with the RAMC in Malta in 1917 but was recruited again to serve during the last two months of 1918, when the spread of influenza meant that thousands of ailing soldiers were admitted to the military hospitals. She worked at the Cambridge Military Hospital at Aldershot, a two-hour train trip from her home in London, and where Phoebe Chapple had worked in her first military appointment in 1917. Close by to the Cambridge Military Hospital is the Aldershot Military Cemetery. It contains ninety graves of soldiers who died after the Armistice and bears witness to the Spanish influenza's fatal ability well into 1919.

There was often little that the doctors and the nurses could do to combat the ravages of influenza. Sister Elsie Tranter from Melbourne, working in the influenza ward in an Abbeville hospital, recorded in her journal that she was afraid that three of her patients would die before the morning. In February 1919 she wrote of influenza: 'This is a cruel disease. No matter how hard we work or what we do for the boys, the germ seems to get stronger and the boys succumb. Surely they have suffered enough already.'[25]

At the Endell Street Military Hospital in London, Vera Scantlebury wrote in the last week of October 1918 that the rush was still on, there was no breathing space and they had 'heaps of flu and some very sick men'.[26] A week later she recorded an abominable day. One of her 'men' had died and

> the flu cases rolling in, eleven of the orderlies lying in H ward not caring one atom about who won the war or anything else . . . the last half mile of the race is always the hardest.[27]

Western Front: Étaples, France

November 1918, Autumn
At the 46th Hospital in Étaples, the end of the war in November 1918 and the ensuing demobilisation severely depleted the staff numbers, but Marjory stayed. The influenza epidemic meant that the hospital was still full, and the demand for diagnostic services continued unabated. She worked on in her laboratory well into 1919. Later that year, Marjory finally decided it was time to go home and in December she boarded the SS *Indarra*. This was fortunate because before being requisitioned as a troopship by the Australian government in late 1917, the ship was a coastal trader owned by the Australian Steam Navigation Company. At the time, the *Indarra* had been the most opulent liner serving along the Australian coast, with a marble open-air swimming pool and a lift between decks. However, the boat's design problems gave it

a heavy roll, which Marjory and all the passengers experienced as they crossed the Great Australian Bight. A committee of passengers also complained about overcrowding, poor food and service but the ship duly arrived in Sydney on 5 February 1920.[28]

The *Indarra* brought home Marjory and also Australian painter Lieutenant Arthur Streeton who, after a year with the RAMC, had been engaged by the Australian government as a war artist.[29] While Marjory was working in her Étaples laboratory, Streeton had been painting scenes of the war around Amiens and Boulogne, 7 kilometres away. Marjory returned to a position as demonstrator in pathology at the University of Sydney and opened a private pathology practice. In 1923 she published her work on bacillary and amoebic dysentery in the *Medical Journal of Australia*, based on her wartime experiences in Rouen and Étaples.[30]

Chapter 8

'By Gosh! It's Peace!'[1]

Orderly at Endell Street Military Hospital, London, 11 November, 1918

At 11 am on 11 November 1918, Agnes Bennett was on a train. When the North Eastern pulled into Doncaster Station in Yorkshire, dramatic news reached the passengers. The war was over. Arriving in London, Agnes saw that everyone was out on the streets, many in celebratory tears. All work was abandoned and the windows were full of flags.

A little while later, Agnes was reunited with one of her brothers and they stood in the huge, joyous crowd outside Buckingham Palace swelling the chorus of 'We want Queen Mary' and 'We want King George' until the royal couple emerged.[2] The guns had been silenced but the work of military hospitals continued apace and the following day, Agnes departed for the Welsh Military Hospital at Netley on Southampton Water.

In the operating theatre of the Endell Street Military Hospital in London, Vera Scantlebury was just completing a lengthy operation when she heard the maroons, the cannons used to warn of air-raids, boom three times at 11 am.

'There was an electric thrill thro' all of us as we gazed at each other and incredulous smiles dawned on our faces. Then an orderly exclaimed waving a swab in her hand "By Gosh! It's Peace!" We could not believe it.'[3]

Paddy and Garrett, the OC's dogs, tore round and round the hospital's courtyard, barking madly as the orderlies and patients cheered and the piano struck up song after song. A convoy of wounded had come in at midnight and Vera had another operation to complete, but at midday she was able to head out into London's packed streets. One young man clapped her on the back and said 'And hurrah for nursie' and another asked 'What are you going to do now the war is over?' Vera wrote that it was only 12.30! After a day of celebration 'the hospital goes on as usual and never have we been more busy'.[4]

Vera wrote that it was the most wonderful day in all history but she also said that she felt very flat and numb. An RAMC friend agreed; many of his colleagues felt dazed and were not sure whether to go to church or get drunk. Within days of the Armistice, there was a general feeling of unrest at the hospital. There was work to do but everyone was unsettled and wondering what would come next.

> Our past lives – 'before the war' – slip from our memory like reality from the minds of those that dream. Our future – 'when the war is over' – the mind refuses to grasp. There seems no other life.[5]

The lives of the women doctors during the war years had become their normal way of living and of practising their profession, and they were acclaimed by the press: 'They really do splendid work!' (*Auckland Star*, 16 May 1917); 'they are our own women who have been doing such splendid work' (*Melbourne Punch*,

24 January 1918); 'such splendid work in the military hospitals' (*The Australasian*, 9 February 1918).

But with the end of hostilities, everything had to be renegotiated. Despite their war service, which demonstrated that women doctors could exercise the same professional skills as their male colleagues, the post-war period saw a return to the exclusion of women from what Dr Flora Murray called 'the professional prizes' in medicine.[6] Vera had anticipated this when she wrote to a friend in October 1917 that 'my work will not count afterwards by way of experience', a prescience that proved to be quite accurate.

What happened to the professional lives of the women featured in this book immediately after the war and into the 1920s? Laura Forster had died in Galicia in January 1917. Lillias Hamilton, Irene Eaton and Eveline Benjamin Cohen all died in the 1920s, the latter two at a relatively young age. Before the war, women doctors were marginalised into the public health sector: school and council inspections, asylums and dispensaries. After the war, little changed. Letitia Fairfield returned to her position as senior medical officer with the London City Council, working there until 1948 except for the period of her enlistment during World War II. Eleanor Bourne became assistant medical officer for the City of Carlisle in north-west England and did not return home to Brisbane until 1937. Both Letitia's and Eleanor's positions were primarily concerned with child and maternal welfare. Isabel Ormiston was appointed as the Senior Lady Medical Officer in the Egyptian Ministry of Education and, dating her career from 1913, remained overseas for thirty-six years.

Elizabeth Hamilton-Browne's professional life also occurred overseas – in India. The life and culture of the East attracted Elizabeth, and at the end of the war she accepted a one-year position in India on the staff of the Surgeon General of the Punjab.

She then remained in India for twenty years,[7] holding several positions in Calcutta, New Delhi and Lahore. In 1941 she became Lady Assistant to the Inspector-General of Civic Hospitals in the Punjab. Elizabeth retired to Australia in 1952, living to 102 years of age.

Of those who returned home and worked in public health in Australia, Hilda Bull Esson became a medical officer with the Melbourne City Council and Isabella Younger Ross worked voluntarily to pioneer baby health centres in Victoria on her return from England in 1917.

Vera Scantlebury sought an honorary consultant position at Melbourne's Children's Hospital for six years in order to gain a foothold in the developing specialty of paediatrics. In 1925 she gave up in despair, having been continually blocked in her goal to become a children's medical practitioner, and a year later accepted the position in Victoria's Department of Public Health as the first Director of Infant Welfare.

Emma Buckley and Marjory Little arrived back in Sydney in 1919 and continued to work in the field of pathology. Emma was appointed as pathologist at the Royal North Shore Hospital and Marjory developed her own very successful private pathology practice.

Elsie Dalyell returned to London from her work with the RAMC on the cholera epidemic in Constantinople in 1919. She was immediately asked, along with Dr (Dame) Harriette Chick, to lead a study team from the Lister Institute and the United Kingdom Medical Research Council that was going to Vienna. The medical team was to study the role of nutrition in the prevalence of rickets in Viennese children after the war.

Between 1919 and 1922, Elsie was the senior clinician in the team that researched the disease of rickets; this research was a major landmark in the discovery of the relationship between rickets, vitamins and ultraviolet light.[8] The two doctors published their findings in scientific papers in both English and German, and the Lister Institute prevailed upon Elsie to remain in London. However, Elsie had been away from Australia for almost ten years and felt she should contribute her expertise to the health system at home.

She left England in March 1923, undertaking a lecture tour in America on the findings of the Viennese study on her way home to Australia. The best that Australia could offer was a position as an assistant microbiologist in the Department of Public Health in Sydney. Routine laboratory tests and no real possibility for advancement became Elsie's career prospects.

Lucy Gullett, Agnes Bennett, Phoebe Chapple and Lilian Cooper returned to their pre-war medical practices and the daily routine of patients, home visits and work in maternity hospitals. Agnes Bennett found that it was not at all easy to settle down and that she needed to cultivate a new perspective on life and her profession.

Katie Ardill and Mary De Garis both started anew. Katie established a gynaecological practice in Sydney and, with Lucy Gullett, worked to found Sydney's Rachel Forster Hospital for Women and Children. Mary settled in the Victorian country town of Geelong, setting up a practice as an obstetrician and working for the establishment of a maternity ward, with antenatal and postnatal clinics, at the new Geelong Hospital.

After the war, none of the Australian women doctors who had acted as surgeons between 1914 and 1919 pursued a predominantly surgical career, other than in obstetrics, and certainly not in general and orthopaedic surgery.[9] Of course this begs the question of their desire to do so and there is little evidence of their post-war intentions. But Dr Isabel Emslie, who took over command of the SWH unit at Ostrovo after Mary De Garis' departure, wrote that the happiest time of her professional life was when she worked as a surgeon with the SWH in Serbia. However, she also 'knew that it would be unwise and unprofitable to make surgery my life's work at Home' and that she would get nowhere by trying.[10]

In the war's aftermath, the experience and accomplishments of these women received little recognition and both social and professional expectations of the role of women doctors returned to those of pre-war. Nevertheless, doctors like Elsie Dalyell, whose considerable expertise was honed in her wartime laboratories, contributed hugely to the health of Australian families for many generations.

Officially prevented from enlisting and denied gazetted commissions, women doctors were further disadvantaged post-war. Unlike their enlisted male colleagues, they could not remain on army pay while completing further professional qualifications, and while a few were financially independent, most needed to earn their living once their wartime work was completed. With no official enlistment, they could not benefit from government legislation that gave employment preference to returned servicemen and neither could they seek a pension for any ill health resulting from their war work.

Over the course of the Great War, there was really no type of surgery or medical procedure that a woman doctor could not perform. For the first time, women doctors treated male patients, took charge of laboratories and published hospital-based scientific papers. Australian women doctors served in at least twelve countries and travelled thousands of kilometres on steam ships, barges, trains, buses, ambulances, sleds and on horseback. They worked in large cities, in ancient abbeys, in converted grand hotels and in tents kilometres from the nearest town. Some came under fire, two were made prisoners of war and one never came home. Influenza, malaria and trauma took a toll on their health throughout their lives.

Many of their male colleagues rightfully gained considerable professional advancement as a result of their war service, which often reinforced their pre-war networks. However, for the women doctors, wherever they went after the war, they faced restricted and gendered choices regarding their professional lives. When war once more engulfed the world in 1939, the enlistment of women doctors with the Australian army for overseas service was again rejected. The only two Australian women known to have done so were Major (Dr) Mary Thornton (Kent Hughes) and Dr Isabel Ormiston. Mary went to London in February 1940 to join the RAMC and served as a radiologist in the Middle East.[11] Isabel was still working at her post–World War I position in Egypt and worked as an anaesthetist in a Cairo military hospital during the Second World War.

In May 1958, Marjory Little was the first woman invited to give the annual Postgraduate Oration in the Great Hall of the University of Sydney. She wrote the speech sitting at her desk overlooking her beautiful garden with its lavender hedges, stone terraces, willows and cherry trees.[12] Of the women who had pioneered the entry of women into medicine and those who had gone to war, she said that they

> were well aware of the responsibilities they accepted in the demanding profession of medicine. Personal success was associated in their minds with recognition of what such successes might mean, not only to themselves, but to those who were to follow them. That they did not fail has placed all

medical women . . . in their debt – a debt which can best be repaid through the years by the maintenance of the standard they set.[13]

The women doctors who went to the Great War had taken part in an event that was central to the lives of their generation. Despite the lack of opportunity after the war, their participation had given them incredible experience of personal autonomy and a new confidence in their professional abilities. Their legacy was to provide another stepping stone towards the acceptance of women into the medical profession and, eventually, should they desire, onto the battlefield. The 'lady doctor' had been redefined.

Biographical notes

Dr Katie Louisa Ardill (Brice)

1886–1955

Born in 1886 in Sydney, Katie Louisa was the first child of George Ardill and British born Louisa Wales. Katie had a younger brother, George Edward, born in 1889. Both of her parents were energetic Baptist social workers and evangelists who were very active in improving the social and medical support for poor women and children of Sydney. They devoted their lives to a wide range of reformist charity organisations.

Katie attended Wellesley College in Newtown and, with the example of her mother's hospital administration work in establishing the South Sydney Women's Hospital, she enrolled in medicine in 1908 and graduated in 1913 from the University of Sydney MB, ChM. She was then appointed to a year's residency at Royal Prince Alfred Hospital, Sydney – a high honour – and became an honorary anaesthetist and out-patients' medical officer at South Sydney Women's Hospital.

In 1914, when World War I began, Katie was twenty-eight years old. Although she wanted to contribute to the war effort, she was rejected by the Australian military when she tried to enlist. Instead she departed for London on 26 June 1915 where she offered her services to the British Red Cross Society. She was accepted immediately and deployed to Calais on the French coast, where she served at the Anglo–Belgian Hospital from September 1915 to February 1916.

In mid-1916 the British army allowed women doctors to be 'enlisted' on a contractual basis and ex-officio capacity and Katie joined the RAMC. She worked at the County of Middlesex War Hospital at Napsbury, England, till January 1917; the Dover Military Hospital until May 1918; and the Citadel Hospital, Cairo, with the army of occupation into 1919.

She was recalled to England in mid-1919 and repatriated home to Sydney by October of the same year. For her services she was awarded the British Red Cross Medal.

The following year Katie resumed her hospital appointment at the Women's Hospital in Newtown, south Sydney, where she continued to work until 1950. She also set up her own private practice in gynaecology in Macquarie Street, Sydney, as well as providing a regular free clinic for servicemen's wives and children. She married Charles Christie Brice, a law student and later accountant, at St Andrew's Cathedral in Sydney's heart on 1 June 1921.

A spirited and energetic person, who 'smoked perennially', Katie was a very active volunteer. She was a member of the St John Ambulance Brigade and served on the brigade's executive committee from 1938, becoming deputy chair in 1947 to 1948 and their first woman chair from 1950 to 1955. Recognised with an OBE in 1941, she was also made a sister of the Order of St John of Jerusalem in 1938 and Dame of Grace of the order in 1952.[1]

In 1952, at the age of sixty-six, she travelled to London to study the latest treatments for victims of atomic blasts, particularly relevant to St John as a medical emergency organisation. Three years later she died in St Luke's Hospital, Sydney, on 3 January 1955 aged sixty-nine; her funeral service was held at St Andrew's Church of England, Roseville.

Dr Ethel Mary Dorothea Nevill Baker

1885–1965

Ethel was born at Toowong just outside Brisbane, Queensland, in 1885 to parents John Hamilton Baker, aged thirty, an architect and surveyor, and Ethel Jemina Nevill née Perkins, aged twenty-nine. Ethel Jemina had spent part of her childhood in Bengal, India, where her father was a colonel with the British army. John and Ethel emigrated from England to the colony of Queensland in 1884 to start a new life away from Ethel's family, who believed she had married beneath her class.[2] They lived on Sylvan Road in Toowong near the Brisbane River. Tragically, in 1886 when baby Ethel was just six months old, her mother died.[3]

A handwritten embarkation list for the SS *Garth Castle* shows that Ethel was ten years old when she travelled to England as an 'unaccompanied' child and arrived in London on 19 June 1894 via Durban, South Africa. Her father had remarried and her new stepmother failed to bond with his child. Ethel was sent to live with her mother's family in West Kensington and then to her grandparents' home on the Isle of Wight. The *Garth Castle* later became one of His Majesty's Hospital Ships with 250 beds and stood by at Gallipoli.

It is not known where Ethel was educated or when she made the decision to study medicine in Brussels, Belgium. Evidently there was family money to sponsor her university education.

Ethel moved to Belgium in 1908, aged twenty-two, and lived with relatives at 13 Rue Africaine, Brussels, an area of narrow streets with attractive brick and stucco three-storey buildings and wrought-iron Juliet balconies. The house was a convenient fifteen-minute walk to the prestigious University of Brussels and its medical school, which admitted women students. From

1908 to 1913, Ethel studied medicine at the university; its reputation attracted enrolments from all around the world.

She graduated in 1913 but Ethel still had to complete the
LMSSA to qualify for registration in Britain. She passed the
examination in London and was registered as a medical practitioner on 2 February 1914.

With the outbreak of World War I that same year, Ethel's
half-brother, Richard Hamilton Baker, joined the AIF in the first
weeks but died in the initial assault on Gaba Tepe at Gallipoli on
25 April 1915. Missing in action, his body was never recovered.[4]

Records about Ethel's war service are scant but in 1914 she
joined the BFH, which established its hospital at 99 Boulevard
Leopold, Antwerp. She was registered with the Belgian Red
Cross in late September of 1914 and issued with her official *bras-
sard*, or armband, to underline her status as a *Docteur*. In Belgium,
she worked with Australian Dr Laura Forster and two English
women doctors, under Dr J Hartnell Beavis. In September and
October 1914 Belgium was a battle zone as the German army
attacked the cities of Liège and then Antwerp. The medical
staff were evacuated back to London and when Dr Beavis
invited the women doctors to join his new unit at Furness, Ethel
declined.[5] Her war service entitled her to the Victory Medal
and the British War Medal – the same as those awarded to her
brother Richard.

After Antwerp, Ethel worked as a doctor to miners and their
families in Staffordshire and in 1916 she took a position assisting
the first woman doctor at Nottingham in the English Midlands,
becoming the second. She lived at the Old Vicarage, an old stone
building, at the village of Hyson Green, Nottingham.

Ethel was also appointed as a medical officer with the
Nottingham Venereal Disease Clinic and the School Medical

Inspection Service as well as being Honorary Physician for the Collin's Trust Maternity Hospital in Castlegate. This hospital was created in 1915 specifically for unmarried women, and cared for the increased numbers of pregnant single mothers during and after the war. Hyson Green was a very poor area and Ethel treated people whether or not they could afford to pay.

In later life Ethel moved closer to London, to 58 Woodstock Road, Bedford Park, Chiswick, near Hyde Park, living with Dorothy Fisk. Ethel died of a stroke on 12 March 1965 at the age of eighty, in Acton Hospital, London. With no children, Ethel's estate of £30,291 was bequeathed to Dorothy Fisk.

Dr Eveline Rosetta Benjamin (Cohen)

1879–1922

Eveline Rosetta Benjamin was born in central Hobart, Tasmania, in 1879 to parents Fannie and Samuel Benjamin. One of three children, she had a brother and an older sister, Lydia. Her family were early settlers in Tasmania and the Georgian townhouse Temple House on the corner of Argyle and Liverpool Streets, where Eveline lived from 1894 to 1905, was built by her great-uncle Judah Solomon in 1832 at a cost of £500.[6] Eveline's father, Samuel, was a wealthy businessman and prominent figure in the Hobart community, serving as a council alderman and president of the Hobart Hebrew Congregation. He was also well known for his magnificent garden at Temple House and his interest in pigeons.

Eveline attended Presentation College, now St Mary's College, Hobart, and went on to become one of the first Australian Jewish women to graduate in medicine. She studied firstly for a year at the University of Melbourne in 1904 and then enrolled at the Edinburgh College of Medicine for Women from 1905 to 1909. In Edinburgh she excelled, winning various medals, including one for clinical surgery, and gaining her MB. She followed this by completing her FRCS at the University of Dublin in 1910.[7] Her first appointment was to the Manchester Jewish Hospital in England and, following her marriage to Harry Cohen, she took up infant welfare work in 1911. She was appointed as medical officer to the Jewish Infant Welfare Centres in Underwood Street, Cable Street and Dame Collett House in London.

Late in 1914 she convened ambulance and hygiene classes for the British Red Cross Society and the VADs, and in 1915 became the tuberculosis officer at the Brighton Borough Sanitorium – the first woman doctor to hold this position.

The following year, while her husband was serving in France with the London Rifle Brigade,[8] she was contracted for war service as a medical officer with the RAMC at Salonica and Malta military hospitals. She served for a year, completing her contract in Malta in September 1917. Although her health suffered from her time with the RAMC, she volunteered to work for six weeks in late 1918 at the Cambridge Military Hospital, Aldershot, when the influenza epidemic raged. Harry's brigade served in France throughout the war, and he survived his wartime service.

After the war, Eveline returned to part-time work at her previous infant welfare centre in Underwood Street, London. She worked with mothers and babies of the poor East End area of London until January 1920, when she began her last appointment as assistant medical officer for the County of Somerset.[9]

Eveline was made an honorary life member of the British Red Cross Society for her work with VADs during the war. She died in 1922 aged forty-three at Weston-super-Mare in England. Harry and Eveline did not have a family of their own and, from her estate, she bequeathed money to her two nephews to encourage them to study medicine.

Dr Agnes Elizabeth Lloyd Bennett

1872–1960

Agnes Bennett's early childhood was spent at idyllic Shell Cove, Neutral Bay, on Sydney's then rural north shore. Her father, William, an engineer, and her mother, Agnes, purchased a beautiful home named Honda that sat just above the bay. Agnes, their first child, spent much of her time trying to keep up with her two younger brothers, playing in the paddocks in front of the house which led down to the beach. When she was five and a half years old, her mother took the family to England for the children's education and in 1878 Agnes was enrolled at Cheltenham Ladies' College. She was their youngest pupil. The principal, Miss Beale, was a pioneer of women's education and Agnes had powerful female role models in her first three years of schooling.

Tragedy struck the family in 1880 when Agnes' mother died of smallpox; the grieving family returned to their home in Sydney. Agnes dealt with her grief by retreating into books but her new stepmother feared her constant reading, saying that Agnes wanted to know too much. Agnes completed the final years of her secondary schooling at Sydney Girls High School, which was the alma mater of five Australian World War I women doctors: Agnes, Emma Buckley, Elsie Dalyell, Lucy Gullett and Grace Cordingley. Agnes, however, could not afford to study medicine so she studied science instead, graduating Bachelor of Science from the University of Sydney in 1894.

Scientific positions were unavailable to women and so she accepted work as a governess in outback New South Wales. But Agnes was determined to study medicine and she borrowed money to relocate to the Edinburgh College of Medicine for Women in Scotland, graduating MB, ChM in 1899 and MD in 1911. While studying, she formed close female friendships with the other women 'medicals', including her teacher Dr Elsie Inglis, who founded the SWH in 1914, which Agnes would later join.[10]

As a new graduate, Agnes worked at the Larbert Asylum, Scotland, but then returned to Australia where she worked in private practice in Sydney from 1901 to 1904; at the Hospital for the Insane at Callan Park from 1904 to 1905; in private practice in Wellington, New Zealand, from 1905 onwards; and at St Helen's Maternity Hospital, Wellington, from 1908 to 1936 (with the exception of the war years).

When Agnes' brothers enlisted in the Australian military, she also felt a responsibility to serve. Refused enlistment, she was sailing to France via Egypt when she witnessed the Gallipoli wounded being unloaded on the docks in Port Said. Agnes disembarked and served in two hospitals in Cairo for almost a year. She then continued on to London and was almost immediately recruited by the SWH. She went on to establish and lead the SWH's America Unit at Ostrovo (then in northern Macedonia) in 1916 and 1917.

After leaving the SWH and recovering from malaria, Agnes joined a troopship as a medical officer and sailed home to Sydney.[11] The following year she returned to Wellington, New Zealand, until March 1918 when she again decided to assist the war effort. She sailed back to England to visit the SWH headquarters. There she heard that the Glasgow Infirmary needed a medical officer. She worked there for four months, coping with the influenza pandemic as the only doctor at hand.

Agnes resigned, exhausted, but despite the war ending on 11 November went on to work at the Welsh Military Hospital at Netley, on Southampton Water. By Christmas, patient numbers were dwindling and the armed forces were rapidly demobilising. Agnes joined a New Zealand troopship, the *Paparoa*, to sail home. Arriving at Wellington in May 1919, the ship was given a rousing welcome and Agnes felt it reaffirmed her earlier decision that this was where she wanted to settle.[12]

Post-war, Agnes resumed her private practice, mostly in obstetrics and as a consultant to various Wellington hospitals, such as St Helen's Maternity Hospital. She continued to be deeply involved with the community and became the first president of the Wellington branch of the International Federation of University Women in 1923. She regularly attended the British Medical Association conferences, visiting Australia often. As a staunch feminist, she was a public opponent of prominent New Zealand infant welfare proponent Dr Frederic Truby King, who advocated that women's place was in the home.

Seeking adventure again, in 1938 she moved to Burketown, north Queensland, as medical officer at the base hospital for the Flying Doctor Service. With the outbreak of World War II she returned to Wellington and helped to form the Women's War Service Auxiliary. She then sailed to London and worked in hospitals from 1940 to 1942 before finally returning to New Zealand at the age of seventy.

Over her life, Agnes Bennett contributed greatly to the improvement of maternal and infant medical care in New Zealand, and did much to advance women's status. For these contributions she was awarded an OBE in 1948. In 1955 and 1956 she donated £10,000 for aeronautical research to the University of Sydney, and she died three years later in Wellington on 27 November 1960.

Dr Eleanor Elizabeth Bourne

1878–1957

Eleanor Elizabeth Bourne was the first woman to graduate in medicine in Queensland, the first woman resident at the Brisbane General Hospital and also the first medical officer in the Queensland Department of Public Instruction, in 1911. Her *Australian Dictionary of Biography* entry describes her as an 'unusually confident and self-reliant woman'.[13]

Born in Brisbane in 1878 the first child of three, her father was John Sumner Bourne, a clerk in the Land Commission Court, and her mother was Jane Elizabeth, née Hocking. Eleanor attended three schools: Leichhardt State School, Brisbane Central School for Girls and Brisbane Girls' Grammar.[14] An outstanding student, in her final year of secondary school, 1896, she won a government exhibition to the University of Sydney – the first ever to be awarded to a woman – and the Grahame & John West Gold Medals for academic achievement. Eleanor continued to win various honours at university and graduated MB, ChM in 1903. Her academic excellence enabled her to obtain a resident medical officer position at the Women's Hospital, Sydney, from 1903 to 1907. She then became the first woman resident at the Brisbane General Hospital and worked also at the Hospital for Sick Children in Brisbane.[15]

Eleanor Bourne began her private practice in Wickham Street, Brisbane, and she also worked as an honorary out-patient physician and anaesthetist at the Children's Hospital. In early 1911 she was appointed to the Queensland Department of Public Instruction as their first medical officer. Believing strongly in the need for public health education, she travelled extensively around outback towns including Charleville, Cunnamulla, Thargomindah, Augathella,

Eulo, Blackall, Longreach and Barcaldine. In 1912 she visited many towns in the north Queensland region, from Mackay up to Cairns.[16] A female doctor travelling independently in outback regions was exceptional at the time. Eleanor also provided research for the hookworm survey of northern Queensland and reported on ophthalmia in western Queensland. Responding to community needs, she published dietary guidelines for parents of school children.

When the war continued on into 1915, Eleanor applied for leave from her government position to offer her services. Travelling to London in early 1916, she was invited to join the Endell Street Military Hospital, where she served as a lieutenant, rising to the rank of major in 1917. She found the experience of working with the senior British suffragette women doctors who had created the hospital very satisfying indeed and also met Mrs Emmeline Pankhurst in London. 'It was indeed a pleasure and an inspiration to be associated with so many splendid women.'[17] In late 1917, Eleanor was appointed as a medical officer to QMAAC.

After the war, Eleanor remained in England and obtained her Diploma of Public Health in 1920. She was appointed as the assistant medical officer for the City of Carlisle in north-west England, organising a new maternity hospital and the child and maternal services. In 1928 she applied for the position of the Commonwealth Director of Maternal Hygiene and Children's Welfare in Australia. When offered far less than the male equivalent salary, Eleanor queried this and when equivalence was not forthcoming she refused the position.

Eleanor did not return to Australia until 1937, an absence of more than twenty years. She never married but returned at the age of fifty-nine to settle in Manly, Sydney.

For her services she was made an honorary life member of the British Medical Association.

From 1914 Eleanor's family had been closely involved with the development of the Women's College at the University of Queensland and the college named a wing in her honour. She served as a vice president of their standing committee and later donated £1000 to the college. She died in 1957, aged seventy-nine years.[18]

Dr Emma Albani Buckley (Turkington)

1879–1959

Emma Albani Buckley was born in Batley, Yorkshire, in 1879, to parents George Buckley, a musician, and his wife, Alice Pulleine. The family emigrated to Sydney and Emma attended Sydney Girls High School, then commenced a Bachelor of Science at the University of Adelaide.[19] She decided to study medicine at the University of Sydney and began living at the Women's College. Working as a governess and school teacher to earn money for her studies, she graduated MB, ChM in 1911.[20]

Emma was a talented pathologist and in 1915 carried a letter of introduction to the Lister Institute of Preventive Medicine in London where she hoped to contribute to the war effort. She received a Jenner Research Scholarship for one year and spent the subsequent war years in London, working for a short period at the Endell Street Military Hospital but mostly in the pathology department of the King George Military Hospital.

Emma returned to Sydney in early 1919 where, during the influenza epidemic, she took charge of the Red Cross influenza depots. She was appointed to the position of medical super-intendent of Royal North Shore Hospital from January 1920 until

December 1921 and also worked at the Rachel Forster Hospital. In 1923 she was appointed medical officer to hat-makers Jones Brothers Limited, and in 1925 was president of the Professional Women Workers' Association. Emma remained a committed feminist throughout her life.

Emma married Samuel Turkington in 1922 and they moved to New Zealand late in 1925. In Auckland she became a prominent activist in women's affairs, working through the Federation of University Women and as medical adviser to the National Council of Women. In 1932–1933 Emma toured England, Europe and the United States and made a special study of child guidance, a new system in managing child behaviour and emotional problems recently inaugurated in the United States and operating in many cities in England. She also attended the international conference of the British National Council of Women.[21] Emma Turkington died in Fulham, London, in 1959.

Dr Hilda Wager Bull (Esson, Dale)

1886–1953

Hilda Wager Bull was born in 1886 in the Sydney suburb of Waverley; her mother was Kate Marina Harris and her father, Thomas William Bull, was a successful herbalist. Thomas wanted all of his children – Hilda, Lionel, Noel and Vivienne – to study medicine and Hilda and Noel obliged.

The family soon moved to Melbourne, living in Armadale initially, where Hilda attended the local primary school and made a lifelong friend in the writer Katherine Susannah Pritchard. The family then moved to a rambling brick and stone house called Orme Hurst in Ormond in Melbourne's south-east. Always a forceful personality, Hilda made the decision to be educated at the Presbyterian Ladies' College, Kew, finding another good friend in Nettie Higgins (Palmer). Hilda matriculated in March 1906 and completed a medical degree, MB, ChB with distinction at the University of Melbourne in 1913.

At the university she was exposed to a rich cultural milieu of alternative ideas, particularly as a foundation member of the Melbourne University Dramatic Society. It was here that she met Louis Esson, poet and playwright. After working for a time as a medical practitioner, she and Louis were married in December 1913 in Melbourne by radical clergyman Dr Charles Strong of the Australian Church. This was Esson's second marriage and he had a son, Jimmie. Hilda was described as 'a gifted, strong-minded woman with broad interests. Her economic, intellectual and emotional support enabled Louis to pursue his career as a dramatist and freelance writer at a time when writing was a poorly rewarded and disheartening pursuit.'[22]

Hilda and Louis left Melbourne for America in late 1916 with the intention of promoting Louis' plays in New York. But due to a lack of success and their dislike of the American culture of New York, they moved to London in late 1917, where they settled in Bloomsbury.

Louis had been rejected by the Australian army but Hilda soon found medical war work and was employed by the WAAC as a member of a travelling medical board, where she examined the women army recruits. A trailblazer as a professional doctor and working mother, she bore her only child, Hugh Thomas Esson, in 1918 and returned to her medical work for the WAAC some months later. Although childcare was provided by a neighbour and her husband, Louis, she found her double load exhausting and contracted pneumonia the following year.[23]

Hilda and her family returned to Melbourne in 1921 and she continued to support her husband and his career. Their friendship with Vance and Nettie Palmer produced the Pioneer Players, a theatre group dedicated to performing Australian plays in which Hilda often acted.[24]

Hilda was appointed medical officer to the Melbourne City Council, where she worked for the next twenty-three years. In 1927 she became assistant to Dr John Dale, health officer to the City of Melbourne. Louis Esson died in 1943 and Hilda continued to work until her retirement, due to ill health, in 1950. Her work was publicly acknowledged in *The Argus*: 'deaths from diphtheria dropped from 14 a year to none' and 'she earned world fame for her research into poliomyelitis.'[25]

In 1951 Hilda married John Dale and they travelled to Italy but John Dale was killed in a car accident near Venice and Hilda was badly injured. Hilda's health never fully recovered and she died in Melbourne in June 1953 aged sixty-seven.

Dr Rachel Champion (Shaw)

1890–1965

Rachel Champion was born in Melbourne in 1890 to Alfred Champion and his wife, Rachael Patterson.[26] She was educated at Milverton Private Girls' School in Camberwell, a leafy eastern suburb. Qualifying for entrance to the University of Melbourne, she chose to enrol in medicine in 1908. After a slow start, she achieved excellent results in her final year, 1913, and was awarded equal first place, sharing the Fulton Scholarship in Obstetrics and Gynaecology. She also received first class honours in surgery and clinical surgery, winning a P&O scholarship for further study in England.[27] She graduated MB, ChB in early 1914 alongside Dr Vera Scantlebury.

Close friends with Vera, Rachel also met Dr Charles Gordon Shaw at the university; he was one of her tutors and would become her husband in 1917. After graduation she was appointed resident medical officer at St Vincent's Hospital, Melbourne, where Dr Shaw had been appointed as a surgeon the previous year. Rachel completed her appointment in 1915 and in November she sailed to London to offer her services to the Endell Street Military Hospital. She was appointed to the ex-officio rank of captain. Vera started at the same hospital the following year and wrote: 'Hamilton Brown [sic] and Ray are especially good surgeons.'[28] For a short period before her marriage, Rachel moved to a room in the house where Vera lived and they enjoyed watching the Zeppelins passing overhead from Vera's attic room.

In August 1917 Rachel's wedding was delayed when she had her appendix removed, but by October she was well enough to be married to Lieutenant Colonel Shaw in All Soul's Church, at Langham Place, London. Rachel's career at Endell Street Hospital ended when she moved away with her husband, who had been posted to the No. 1 Australian Auxiliary Hospital at Harefield Park in Middlesex – a convalescent hospital for wounded Australians. She visited her friends in London frequently and took on short periods of relief work with the WAAC.

Rachel and her husband had their first child in England in January 1919 and the Shaws sailed back to Melbourne in April that year. Gordon Shaw became an honorary surgeon at St Vincent's Hospital. Rachel raised four children – Michael, Marjorie, Richard and Gordon – and died in 1965, two years before her husband.

Dr Phoebe Chapple

1879–1967

Dr Phoebe Chapple has the honour of being the first Australian woman doctor to win the Military Medal in World War I. Born in 1879 in Adelaide, South Australia, Phoebe was the youngest daughter of a middle-class family of four sons and four daughters. Five of her siblings went on to achieve university degrees. Her parents were Frederic and Elizabeth Chapple Hunter, who were both trained teachers and migrated to Adelaide from Britain in 1876 for Frederic to take up the position of headmaster at Adelaide's prestigious Prince Alfred College for boys.[29]

Phoebe attended the Advanced School for Girls, later known as Adelaide Girls' High School, and completed her schooling at the age of sixteen. She then undertook a Bachelor of Science at the University of Adelaide as she was thought to be too young to study medicine and she graduated in 1898. Phoebe then began her medical training, living in St Anne's College and graduating MB, BS, in 1904 from the University of Adelaide. In 1905 she worked as a house surgeon at the Adelaide Hospital and adventurously left home to work at the Sydney Medical Mission. Returning to Adelaide, she practised from her father's school, the Prince Alfred College, living on the premises and also looking after the health of the student boarders.

She quickly became actively involved in women's issues, gaining a seat on the committee of the South Australian [Women's] Refuge in November 1912. From 1914 to 1929, apart from her war service years, she was honorary medical superintendent of McBride's Maternity Hospital. She was also honorary doctor at the Salvation Army Maternity Hospital for Unmarried Mothers from 1910 to 1940, interrupted only by her war service.[30]

Rejected by the AAMC, she travelled independently to London to join the WAAC instead and was appointed as a surgeon to the Cambridge Military Hospital, Aldershot. She described this as a 'tremendous experience . . . The convoys arrived continually from France and more than 1000 patients were accommodated.'[31]

Phoebe was sent to Abbeville, France, where she came under fire, and for 'gallantry and devotion to duty . . . in the field under fire', she was awarded the Military Medal by the British government. Returning to Adelaide in September 1919, after two and a half years away, she was interviewed by the press, revealing her direct speaking and her modesty: 'Personally, I detest talking of myself, but I had better tell you and be done with it.' Asked when she planned to resume her private medical practice she replied characteristically: 'Straight away . . . I shall begin this week.'[32]

With a passion for assertive feminist political action, Phoebe stood as a candidate in Adelaide's municipal elections in December 1919, supported by the Women's Non-Party Association, but was unsuccessful. She became a founding member and later president of the South Australian Medical Women's Society. From 1921 to 1922 Phoebe was also honorary medical officer in the night clinic at Adelaide Hospital and treated women for venereal diseases.

Phoebe commemorated the Great War by marching every year, leading the nurses' units in the Anzac marches – there was no category for World War I women doctors. She never married or had children and in her later years she made six lengthy trips overseas, maintaining her connections. The British did not forget her heroic war service and in 1937 she was invited to represent South Australia at the coronation of King George VI in Westminster Abbey. She also attended the Medical Women's International Association Conference in Edinburgh and visited Berlin, Vienna and Budapest.

Phoebe continued to conduct her private practice from her

home in Norwood up to the age of eighty-five, dying three years later in 1967. She was honoured at her funeral by the Australian government, who farewelled her with full military honours. In her will, she funded a bursary at the University of Adelaide's St Anne's College and is also commemorated with an annual Phoebe Chapple Memorial PhD Scholarship, awarded by the Australian Medical Women's Memorial Research Fund.

Dr Lilian Violet Cooper

1861–1947

Lilian Violet Cooper, although British by birth, emigrated to Brisbane at the age of thirty with her friend Miss Josephine Bedford in May 1891. She became the first woman doctor registered in the state of Queensland in that same year and worked there for close to fifty-six years; thus she is considered 'Australian' for this book.

Lilian Cooper's decision to emigrate was the first of a number of bold decisions by an adventurous and determined spirit who was able to transcend society's gendered expectations throughout her life. Her Edwardian appearance was also distinctive. She was tall and angular with auburn hair pulled back over high-necked cream shirts and long skirts, but shocked her contemporaries with her brusque manner and colourful language.[33]

Lilian was born in England in Chatham, Kent, the third child of Elizabeth Shewell and Lieutenant Colonel Henry Fallowfield Cooper.[34] She enjoyed a middle-class family life and was educated privately. She was determined to study medicine, against her mother's wishes, and, tutored by two of her brothers, she was accepted at the age of twenty-four by the LSMW. She studied there from 1886 to 1890 completing her MB, ChM and passing the conjoint examinations of the Royal College of Physicians, and the Royal College of Surgeons in Edinburgh and also the Faculty of Physicians and Surgeons in Glasgow, achieving her Licentiate from Edinburgh.[35]

In her first job Lilian worked extremely hard for six months travelling on both horseback and on foot as the first woman to work as a doctor's assistant in England. She wanted to improve her position and, through Dr Elizabeth Garrett Anderson, she successfully applied for a position with a doctor in Brisbane. She and Josephine Bedford, who had become friends during Lilian's medical studies, sailed on the RMS *Lusitania*, reaching Brisbane in May 1891.[36]

Lilian had an unfortunate start to her medical work, encountering obstacles and prejudice. Despite this, she began private practice in Brisbane in December 1891. She was the first woman to be accepted as a member of the Medical Society of Queensland in 1893 and in 1896 she was appointed an honorary medical officer to the Hospital for Sick Children, the first woman in Australia to do so, and to the Lady Lamington Hospital for Women.[37] In 1905 she began a lifelong association with the Mater Misericordiae Hospital, Brisbane.[38]

As with many other single professional Australian women, Lilian decided to travel to London in 1904 and again in 1911 where she could visit her family, witness the women's suffrage campaigns and further her professional learning. During both her trips she visited America and in 1911 she visited the Johns Hopkins Hospital in Maryland and the Mayo Clinic in Rochester, Minnesota. In England in 1912 she successfully sat the examinations to complete her MD from the University of Durham.[39]

After observing World War I from afar for eighteen months, Lilian decided that she should contribute her medical skills and, with the very practical Miss Bedford, she sailed again to London in mid-1916. They were accepted by the SWH and posted to Ostrovo, northern Macedonia, on the Eastern Front to work with Dr Agnes Bennett and Dr Mary De Garis in a 200-bed tented military hospital. They lived in very tough conditions for a year before Lilian's health gave out and she became ill with pneumonia. In mid-August 1917 they sailed to London to recuperate and returned home to Brisbane. For her bravery Lilian was awarded the Medal of St Sava, 4th Class, by the Serbian King and Josephine the Medal of St Sava, 5th Class.

By May 1918 Lilian Cooper had resumed her private practice in Brisbane.[40] A keen cyclist, she was also an early female car owner, driving an Oldsmobile around Brisbane, with Miss Bedford often employing her handy mechanical skills to repair it. A contemporary male doctor described Lilian:

> As a surgeon the doctor displays a skill, a coolness, and a celerity which is not readily understood by those who have not yet learnt that some women can on emergency summon up a nervous force and will-power above that of the other sex. She is equally as successful in large and important surgical operations as in those of a minor character.[41]

In 1923 Lilian was the defendant in a patient's litigation case. The Queensland medical profession and the British Medical Association showed how much they respected her talents by strongly supporting her. She was exonerated and the profession generously contributed money to defray her costs.[42]

Lilian bought the house Old St Marys in 1926 and settled at Kangaroo Point, Brisbane, overlooking the river. She was very active in the Queensland branch of the National Council of Women and in June 1927 became the first woman to be admitted as a Foundation Fellow of the College of Surgeons of Australasia; she was joined by Dr Constance Darcy three months later.[43] She was also a foundation member of the Queensland Medical Women's Society when it began in 1929.[44] Retiring from her medical practice in 1941 at the age of eighty, she died six years later in 1947 and was buried at Toowong Cemetery.

Josephine Bedford donated the house and land to the Anglican Church in 1951 for the Mount Olivet Hospital of the Sisters of Charity, providing a range of care for the sick and elderly, including the Lilian Cooper Nursing Home. There are also memorial windows and an embroidered altar cloth in memory of Lilian at St Mary's Church of England in Kangaroo Point.[45]

Dr Grace Marion Cordingley (Bridge)

1876–1969

Grace Marion Cordingley was born in Grafton, New South Wales, in 1876, one of six children born to Thomas Cordingley and his wife, Jane Susanna Havinden. Thomas was a meat canning technologist and the family moved to Townsville, north Queensland, where he was one of the founders of the North Queensland Meat Export Company, later becoming the managing director.[46] Grace, however, was educated at Sydney Girls High School, where she was prepared for enrolment at the University of Sydney to study Arts. She obtained her Bachelor of Arts in 1898, travelled to Germany and then returned to Sydney to achieve her Master of Arts in 1903 while living at the Women's College.

Grace decided that she wanted to study medicine and sailed with her mother to England to enter the LSMW in the winter of 1903–1904. She was student number 799 and graduated in 1913 at the age of thirty-seven. From June to December that year she was a resident medical officer at the New Hospital for Women in London, founded in 1872 by the first woman to be registered as a physician and surgeon in England, Elizabeth Garrett Anderson.

Grace returned to Australia in 1914 but set out for England again on 24 March 1915 on the SS *Mongolia* and was appointed pathologist to the military section of the Royal Free Hospital, London. She served at the hospital until the Armistice in 1918 and her brother served with the Coldstream Guards regiment.

Grace returned to Australia, leaving England the week after the Armistice in November 1918, on the SS *Balmoral Castle*, which had been used as an Australian troopship, and for part of the way on the SS *Niagara*, travelling home through America. In 1919 she joined a Red Cross team and, with Sydney colleague Dr Emma Buckley, fought the Sydney influenza epidemic.

In early 1920 Grace married an engineer, Reginald Bridge, in Sydney and they had two daughters. She set up her medical practice in Nowra, New South Wales. Grace and Reginald lived on a property called Glen Islay near the little town of Wandanian, south of Nowra, from 1921 to 1935 and later nearby at Milo. In 1929 she attended the British Medical Association's conference in Sydney where she was reunited with many of her medical peers – the women who had served in World War I.[47] She retired from practice in 1956 and died in 1962.

Dr Elsie Jean Dalyell

1881–1948

Members of the Scottish clan Dalyell were early settlers in Australia, arriving soon after the First Fleet. In 1881 Elsie Jean

was born in Newtown, Sydney, to James Dalyell, a mining engineer, and Jean Dalyell (née McGregor). Their second daughter,
Elsie was an exceptionally able student and had no difficulty with
the academic examination for entry to Sydney Girls High School.
The school, designed by convict architect Francis Greenway, was
in the heart of Sydney and Elsie began in 1893 during the prin-
cipalship of Lucy Walker Garvin. The principal had a forceful
personality and expressed high expectations of her female
students; her broad outlook included the belief that girls should
be prepared for university entrance.

In 1897 Elsie joined the Department of Public Instruction as
a student teacher. The department sponsored her to study Arts
and science at the University of Sydney, which she completed in
a single year in 1904. Studying biology became her passion as she
wanted to know much more about the bacteriology of the human
body. She transferred to the medical course and, residing at the
Women's College, she graduated MB in 1909 and ChM in 1910
with first class honours.[48] She completed her residency at Royal
Prince Alfred Hospital.

In 1911–1912 she was made senior demonstrator in pathology
under Professor Welch at the University of Sydney medical school,
the first woman to be appointed to the position and a recognition
of her expertise. She also held honorary pathology positions at
both the Royal Prince Alfred Hospital and the Royal Alexandra
Hospital for Children. In December 1912 Elsie became the first
Australian woman to win a prestigious Beit Fellowship, which she
took up at the Lister Institute of Preventive Medicine, London.
The fellowship provided paid research work for three years and
Elsie studied infantile gastroenteritis, the single biggest cause of
infant mortality in Australia at the time.[49]

Her work at the Lister was disrupted in 1914 when war

was declared and, ever patriotic, she joined the voluntary Lady Wimborne's Serbian Relief Fund field unit in late 1914 and was posted to Serbia from February to July 1915, to contribute her pathology skills to a raging typhus epidemic.

Elsie worked as a pathologist throughout the war in various hospitals: at Addington Park Military Hospital in Croydon, England, from July 1915 to April 1916; at Royaumont Hospital, France, with the SWH from May to October 1916; with the RAMC in Malta from 1916 to 1917; at Salonica's 63rd Hospital from 1917 to 1919; and at Constantinople's 82nd Hospital in 1919. For her services she was 'Mentioned in Dispatches' twice for her bravery and in 1919 awarded an OBE (Military Division).

Arriving back in England from Constantinople, Elsie was immediately recruited to join the Accessory Food Factors Committee as a senior clinician by the British Medical Research Council and the Lister Institute. The team was led by Dr (Dame) Harriette Chick and investigated the effects of vitamin deficiencies in the children of Vienna, where post-war deprivation was affecting their health. The team particularly examined the role of Vitamin D in the prevention of rickets[50] and produced perhaps 'the most complete study of human rickets prophylaxis ever undertaken', finalising their research in 1923.[51]

Elsie had been away from her family in Australia for eleven years and decided to return home in 1923 via America, embarking upon a lecture tour about the Vienna research as she travelled. The British regretted their loss and the Americans would also have liked to retain her knowledge and expertise in their country. Ironically, there was no suitable professional opportunity for her in Sydney. Elsie attempted to establish a private practice in Macquarie Street but, with little capital behind her, the venture did not flourish.[52]

In early 1924 she was working for the government in the Department of Public Health as an assistant microbiologist researching venereal diseases. Many of her contemporaries thought this was 'an inadequate use of a splendid mind and a forceful and most engaging personality'.[53] However, from 1925 to 1935, she contributed her expertise, particularly with all aspects of venereal diseases and prevention, to benefit women and children at the Rachel Forster Hospital. With Dr Maisie Hamilton she opened a venereal diseases clinic at the hospital in 1927. She also lectured in pathology at the University of Sydney medical school – 'a superb teacher with tremendous enthusiasm for her subject'.[54]

Elsie was of fair complexion, with short light-coloured hair and pale blue eyes; she invariably wore practical suits. She never married and eventually shared a house with her sister in Greenwich, Sydney. Her health had suffered from her work and the conditions during the war and she retired in 1946 due to hypertensive arterial disease. Elsie died in November 1948, aged sixty-seven; a woman much loved by her family, friends and colleagues for her infectious sense of humour, her work ethic and sharp intellect. Dr Ann Mitchell has written of her: 'All who knew her agreed that she was one of those rare beings whom it was a privilege to know.'[55] The Dalyell Scholar Scheme at the University of Sydney celebrates her life and is awarded in her name to students who are as exceptional as she was herself.

Dr Mary Clementina De Garis

1881–1963

Mary Clementina De Garis began her life in the outback town of Charlton, in north-west Victoria in 1881. She and her non-identical twin sister, Elizabeth, were the oldest of six siblings. Both of their parents were strong members of the community. Their mother, Elizabeth Buncle, was known for her healing and midwifery skills and Mary's father, Elisha, was a Methodist minister and business entrepreneur in real estate and dried fruit, founding EC De Garis and Co. He was also an influential advocate for irrigation in the dry north-west.[56]

With her sister Elizabeth, Mary moved from Mildura to Melbourne to study at Methodist Ladies' College in 1898 and 1899. She excelled academically and, with her family's encouragement, enrolled to study medicine in 1900 at the University of Melbourne, the thirty-first woman to do so. Graduating MB (1904) and BS (1905), she then went on to become the second woman in the state to achieve her MD in 1907.

The early Melbourne medical women were largely united in their feminist mission to achieve equal rights for women, focusing particularly on a woman's right to knowledge, control and protection of her body. At university the women mentored and tutored each other in the women students' club, known as the Princess Ida Club, created in 1888 as a place where the small number of women attending the university could meet and relax in privacy. Mary also belonged to the Victorian Women Medical Students' Society formed in 1902 when they were prevented from joining the Medical Students' Society. This networking continued throughout their professional lives through the Victorian Medical Women's Society and the British Medical Association, later the Australian Medical Association.

Although Mary did her residency year at the Melbourne Hospital in 1905, the only woman that year, she was philosophically and politically aligned with the medical women at the Queen Victoria Hospital. The hospital was founded in 1896 in the hall of the Welsh Church in La Trobe Street, Melbourne, by Dr Constance Stone to provide medical services for poor women and children, and also clinical experience for women doctors unable to acquire placements in hospitals upon graduation. Mary worked there from 1910 to 1911 as the honorary medical officer to out-patients, then briefly again from 1915 to 1916 and from 1919 to 1922.

Familiar with outback living, Mary took her first paid position at the Muttaburra Hospital, via Rockhampton in north Queensland, from 1906 to 1907 as resident surgeon. Restless and lonely after working in an isolated community for more than twelve months, she travelled for fourteen months, sailing alone to England and America and completing postgraduate courses. She was thrilled to meet the medical women in both countries and to attend the suffrage rallies, hearing the Pankhursts speak in London.

Returning to her family's new home in Sandringham, Melbourne, in 1910, Mary tried to set up in private practice at 24 Collins Street. However, it seemed that people were not yet ready to consult women doctors and the practice failed.

In 1911 she took up a resident surgeon position in Tibooburra Hospital, almost 1600 kilometres from Sydney, in the far north-west corner of New South Wales. In Tibooburra she met Colin Thomson, a farmer, and they were engaged one week before the outbreak of war in 1914.

Mary was patriotic like her father and offered her medical services to the Australian army, but was rejected. Colin volunteered and sailed in 1915 to Egypt, where he was posted to the battle of Gallipoli, then to the Western Front in France as a sergeant. On 4 August 1916 Colin was killed at Pozieres.

A grief-stricken Mary eventually joined the SWH at the end of 1916 and was assigned to the America Unit, based in Ostrovo, northern Macedonia, in early 1917. When the CO, Dr Agnes Bennett, became very ill with malaria and departed in September 1917, Mary was appointed as the CO of the 200-bed tent hospital for twelve months. However, after the unexpected death of her mother, she resigned in September 1918 to travel home to Australia. For her work, she was awarded the Medal of St Sava, 3rd Class, by the grateful Serbian government.

En route to Australia she became ill with Spanish influenza while staying in Rome. Fortunately she was found by two RAMC officers and moved to the American Red Cross Hospital, where she recovered after a long recuperation of six weeks. Mary arrived back in Melbourne in February 1919. By May, she was in Geelong practising as the city's first female medical practitioner and driving her car around Geelong.

Small, with an olive complexion and white hair, Mary's energetic, reformist zeal for women's health helped achieve the election of female members to the Geelong Hospital General Committee in 1925 and the establishment of a dedicated maternity ward, also at the Geelong Hospital, which was commissioned in 1931. That year, she became the head of the new ward, where she established an antenatal and postnatal clinic, bringing 'Melbourne' standards to Geelong. In 1938 the hospital management congratulated her on an exemplary record of 1000 deliveries without the loss of a single mother. Her skill and her mother-focused approach was very popular in Geelong, especially prior to the use of antibiotics and when infant and maternal mortality rates remained a concern.

Mary was also conducting research into the causes of pain in labour; she published approximately forty-eight articles in medical journals. She developed a new definition for labour and did not accept that pain was a necessary part of it; she also discussed uterine inertia, hidden sources of infection such as bad teeth, the effects of diet on pregnancy and particularly toxaemia and other complications of mothers' health. Mary published three books, the most significant being *The Theory of Obstetrics* which was well received in 1931. A hospital matron who worked with Mary in the 1950s wrote, 'Her dietary treatment of toxaemia of pregnancy was revolutionary at the time and became an accepted method in later years.'

Dr Mary De Garis' work at the Geelong Hospital was commemorated with the naming of the hospital's De Garis House. She continued to practise until the age of seventy-nine, as many male doctors did, although this was controversial at the time. Mary died in Geelong in November 1963 from a cerebral haemorrhage and was buried in the Eastern Cemetery. One of her patients said of her, 'She had a mother's natural instincts herself but the whole world was her family.'[57]

Dr Irene Cecil Davy Eaton

1882–1920

Irene Cecil Davy Eaton was born to Henry Francis Eaton and his wife, Elizabeth Davey, in Melbourne, Victoria, in 1882. Henry had emigrated from Nottinghamshire to the gold diggings in 1853, but his career developed with the civil service and by 1889 he had risen to the position of undersecretary of the Victorian State Treasury. He retired from the Treasury in 1895, when Irene was thirteen years old, and he then took the family back to live in England. They lived in a London flat on a rise overlooking Hampstead Heath. Irene was educated privately in Victoria and London and chose to study medicine at the LSMW, graduating MB and ChM in 1909.

Like many women medical graduates, Irene's initial career prospects were limited to public health positions and she obtained an appointment as the medical officer of the East Anglia Sanitorium in Suffolk but later became house surgeon and pathologist at the New Hospital for Women.[58] In 1913 she was appointed assistant health officer to the Willesden Urban Municipal Council in north-east London while also studying for her Diploma of Public Health, which she gained in 1915. Willesden Council was an early municipal leader in London in the provision of maternal and child health centres.

The Eaton family had both family and friends back in Melbourne, and in early 1914 Irene sailed on the SS *Moldavia* to Melbourne for a month-long holiday before returning to the Willesden role and to setting up a practice in the village of Dulwich, England, 20 kilometres to the south.[59]

In the second half of 1916, Irene served at the Norfolk War Hospital as assistant pathologist and then in Malta, attached to the RAMC when they began to offer twelve-month contracts to women doctors. She worked in this position for fourteen months until October 1917 when she returned to England and took a job as a bacteriologist with the WAAC. She was later appointed as Area Controller of QMAAC (formerly WAAC) Eastern Command, where she served until demobilised in June 1919 as the organisation was wound down post-war.

By then almost half of the WAAC members had been demobilised and its services continued to be wound down until it ceased to exist in September 1921. After the war, Irene was one of the first medical officers appointed to Britain's new Ministry of Health. Her colleagues, however, were shocked and saddened when Irene died suddenly of a heart attack on 2 August 1920 at the age of thirty-eight: 'We all loved Dr Eaton – she was so delightful to do with, so ready to help in any difficulty. You could always depend on her . . . always harmonious.'[60]

Dr Josephine Letitia Denny Fairfield

1885–1978

Josephine Letitia Denny Fairfield (known as Letitia) was both Australian and British, being born in St Kilda, Melbourne, in 1885 but moving to the United Kingdom when she was just three years old. She was the eldest of three daughters born to Charles Fairfield, an Irish journalist at the Melbourne newspaper *The Argus*, and Isabella Campbell, of Scottish descent. The family lived in various cities as their father moved jobs frequently. When Letitia was sixteen, her father deserted the family and their mother moved them to Edinburgh to live with family. Letitia and her two sisters were enrolled at George Watson's Ladies' College, which in 1902 became the first prestigious secondary college in Scotland to appoint a female principal.

The move proved fortuitous for Letitia as she wanted to study medicine and, after winning a Carnegie Scholarship and combining that with money from her aunt, she enrolled at the Edinburgh College of Medicine for Women, attached to the University of Edinburgh. She graduated MB, ChB in 1907, gaining honours in all subjects and winning several medals. She worked in various hospital positions to gain clinical experience and was awarded her MD in 1911, again from the University of Edinburgh.[61] She was a passionate feminist and for a short time joined the Women's Social and Political Union but became disillusioned with the Pankhurst leadership.

Relocating with her family to Hampstead, London, Letitia was employed in public health with the London County Council. In 1912, she obtained her Diploma of Public Health from the University of London, specialising in school children's health and welfare including those with disabilities, especially epilepsy. Here she also joined the Fabian Society and was committed to Irish independence. She was a confident public speaker on many health matters.

Letitia offered her services to the British army after war broke out in 1914 but was rejected. Later in 1917 she joined the WAAC as a medical officer and in mid-1918 this was followed by her appointment as a chief medical officer in the Women's Royal Air Force, a new organisation. For her war work, she was awarded the Commander of the British Empire medal.[62]

Post-war Letitia rejoined the London County Council, where she continued to fight for improvements for women and children's health. Letitia also found time to qualify in law as a barrister in 1923 and was a co-editor of the *Medico-Legal and Criminological Review* and president of the Medico-Legal Society in 1957–1958.

During World War II, from 1940 to 1942 she achieved the rank of lieutenant colonel as the Assistant Director-General for Medical Services. After reaching the retirement age of fifty-seven years for the army in 1942, she returned to her previous position with the London City Council and worked for the establishment of the National Health Service in 1948.

Letitia had many varied social and political interests and she helped many Jewish refugees escape Nazi Germany before and during World War II. She had become a Catholic and for her writings for the church she was awarded a Papal Medal in 1965. She did not marry and had a wide extended family; she was described by her peers in the *British Medical Journal* as 'a delightful, dogmatic and at times, infuriating companion'.[63] She died in 1978, aged ninety-two.

Dr Laura Elizabeth Forster

1858–1917

Laura Elizabeth Forster was the daughter of Eliza Wall and William Forster, after whom the town of Forster in New South Wales is named. She was born at the family property Brush Farm House – built by the explorer Gregory Blaxland – on the Parramatta River at Ryde in 1858.[64] Her father was a landowner, member of parliament and Premier of the colony of New South Wales from 1859 to 1860. Laura was the fifth of six children; her mother died in 1862 giving birth to her sixth child and later her father married Maud Julia Edwards. They had five children, including three sons, Laura's half-brothers, who served with the AIF. Sadly all three were killed on active service in France, as well as a cousin.[65]

Laura was educated in Sydney in the years 1864–1876 and after William Forster's death in 1882, she accompanied her stepmother to England. In 1887, Laura entered Bern University's Pathological Institute in Switzerland as a medical student. Graduating in 1894, she was certified to practise medicine in the United Kingdom the following year. Unusually, Laura trained as both a nurse and a doctor and chose to settle in Oxford to practise medicine. She was licensed by the Royal College of Physicians and Surgeons, Glasgow; the Royal College of Physicians, Edinburgh; and the Royal College of Surgeons, Edinburgh.[66]

In 1900 she was appointed medical officer of the Cutler Boulter Dispensary in Oxford. At the outbreak of the First Balkan War in 1912, she travelled to Epirus but served as a nurse because women were not permitted to work as doctors at the battle fronts.[67]

In 1914, with the onset of World War I, Laura immediately joined the BFH and was sent to Belgium. Under bombardment, the staff and patients were evacuated to England but Laura soon returned to another Belgian hospital at La Panne for a short period. In 1915 she made the long journey to Russia, to the largest hospital in Petrograd, where she worked as a surgeon for about a year. With the Russian Red Cross she travelled to the Caucasus; she joined the NUWSS unit working in a district beyond the Volga River at Erzurum, where she was in charge of the hospital. Her final appointment was to Zaleschiki in Galicia to head up the NUWSS hospital established there.[68]

Laura Forster was known as a 'skilful, painstaking and dependable microscopist' and published three articles before World War I in medical journals.[69] But she was also an extraordinarily courageous surgeon and committed feminist. Tragically, in Zaleschiki she contracted influenza and, after a week of illness, she died of heart failure on 29 January 1917.[70] She was described by the administrator of the NUWSS, Miss Moberley, as 'a fair woman with indomitable courage and a love of adventure, which led her to many out-of-the-way corners of the world . . . I believe she was the first English woman ever to work in Petrograd.'[71]

The *Nursing Record* reported her burial with full Russian rites and an open coffin accompanied by icons. The nurses had made a Union Jack which they draped over her coffin. Laura was fifty-eight years old. Her sister donated £500, in 1926, to the University of Sydney's Women's College to establish the Laura Forster Memorial Fund to benefit students of the college.

Dr Laura Margaret Fowler (Hope)

1868–1952

Born in 1868, Laura Margaret Fowler was the first woman to enrol in medicine at the University of Adelaide in South Australia in

1887, graduating in 1891. In that year, she, along with Clara Stone and Margaret Whyte from the University of Melbourne, became the first three women to graduate in medicine in Australia. She was also the first woman doctor to be elected as a member of the British Medical Association, in 1892.[72]

Laura was the second child of Scottish Baptist George Swan Fowler, a very successful wholesale grocer and businessman, and his wife Janet Lamb. Born at Mitcham, south Adelaide, Laura was educated privately in Adelaide, Germany and England. The family lived a comfortable life in South Australia at Wooton Lea House, Glen Osmond, where Laura helped her father to breed leeches for hospitals.[73] The family were committed Baptists and George was president of the Adelaide Baptist Union.

After graduating MB, BS, Laura was offered a residency at the Adelaide Children's Hospital in 1892. She practised medicine for a year and in 1893 married Dr Charles Hope. Feeling a strong vocation to help others, the Hopes set off overseas to East Bengal in India to practise medicine in the missions of the Baptist Church. Over the following two decades they worked at many of the missions, particularly with the South Australian Baptist Mission at Pubna, now in Bangladesh, where they first began their practice. Remaining childless, they were free to devote their lives to this work, which was interrupted only by their service during World War I.

In 1915, the Hopes sailed to London, wanting to assist in the war, and joined the SWH. They were posted to a SWH field unit on the Eastern Front in Serbia. They worked for just four weeks before being taken prisoners of war by the Austrian army and eventually sent to Hungary. After two dreadful months of being regularly shifted, poorly fed and housed, they were released and their unit reached safety in Switzerland in early February 1916.

After recuperating in London from this short but traumatic period of service, the Hopes returned to East Bengal to continue their missionary work at Kalimpong near the border with Bhutan. For their courage, they were both awarded the Serbian Samaritan Cross in 1918 by the Serbian government.

Laura and Charles continued their missionary work, travelling around India, but eventually settled back at Pubna from 1929. The Hopes retired to Adelaide in 1934 and Laura was awarded a further medal – the Kaisar-i-Hind by the British government for public service in India.[74] Laura died in 1952, ten years after the death of Charles, and they lie side by side in Adelaide's Mitcham Cemetery.

Dr Lucy Edith Gullett

1876–1949

Lucy Edith Gullett, the third child of Henry Gullett and Lucy Willie, was born in Hawthorn, Victoria, in 1876. Her father was a journalist and she resembled him: short and with dark hair. Henry relocated the family to Sydney, where Lucy was educated at Sydney Girls High School. In 1901 she became the seventh woman at the University of Sydney to graduate in medicine MB, ChM.

Lucy famously became the first woman resident medical officer at Sydney's Crown Street Women's Hospital and in 1902 was appointed resident surgeon at the Hospital for Sick Children in Brisbane. In 1906, Lucy's father purchased a medical practice for her in the country town of Bathurst. But the town was 200 kilometres north-west of Sydney and she missed her family terribly. After five years she returned home to live with her unmarried sister Minnie in Sydney.[75] The Gullett family were cultural enthusiasts and Lucy and Minnie lived on the shores of Sydney Harbour at Kirribilli.[76]

Towards the end of 1915, Lucy decided to join the voluntary war effort overseas and sailed in 1915 to Cairo, where she worked for some months until the demand for medical services began to decline there. She travelled to London and was immediately recruited to work for the Ulster Volunteer Force Medical and Nursing Corps, which had set up the Hôpital d'Ulster in Lyon. Lucy worked at the hospital throughout 1916, before returning to Sydney at the end of that year. Her efforts for wounded French soldiers were rewarded with the French Red Cross Medal.

In 1919, during the influenza epidemic, she was medical officer at the City Road Emergency Hospital in Sydney. She was honorary out-patient's doctor at the Renwick Hospital for Infants from 1918 to 1932 and a member of the council of the District Nursing Association from 1934 to 1949. As a strong feminist, she worked with Dr Harriet Biffin to found the New South Wales Association of Registered Medical Women in 1921. This was the first step to establishing and funding a women's out-patient clinic that would become the Rachel Forster Hospital for Women and Children, opening in 1925.

Like the Queen Victoria Hospital in Melbourne, the Rachel Forster provided 'care for women by women'.[77] Lucy called the first meeting to inaugurate a committee and contributed much to the hospital as vice-president of the Rachel Forster Committee from 1932 to 1949.[78] She also led the campaign to establish a convalescent home for patients from the Rachel Forster, which was finally built in Bexley in 1946. Those who worked with her said she had 'wisdom and unfailing cheerfulness'.[79] A social worker at the Rachel Forster Hospital, Katharine Ogilvie, wrote:

For twenty-five years she used her wit, her gift of words, her
kindness and her unreasonable optimism to touch the hearts
of women in every walk of life and in every part of Sydney,
so that they became permanent and ardent supporters of the
hospital.[80]

Lucy also had political interests and in 1932 failed in her bid
to enter state politics as an independent. She argued that 'women
had singularly failed to take their place in Australian politics . . .
[although] as legislators for those of their own sex and for children
they could fill a useful place'.[81] A committee member of the United
Associations of Women in 1935, she was vice-president from 1936
to 1938 and again in 1943. Her medical knowledge informed the
association's policies; for example, advocating early marriage as
protection against venereal disease and early divorce where one of
the parties was found to be infected.[82]

Lucy died in her early seventies in 1949 and was buried in the
Gullett family grave at Gore Hill Cemetery in Sydney.

Dr Lillias Anna Hamilton

1858–1925

Lillias Anna Hamilton had a dual identity – an Australian Briton.
Born forty-two years before the Australian colonies federated,
she was the eldest daughter of Englishman Hugh Hamilton and
Margaret Clunes Innes, who was a daughter of George Innes
of Yarrow, New South Wales. When Lillias was still a young
child the family moved back to England and she was educated at
Cheltenham Ladies' College under the guidance of Miss Beale,
who emphasised the importance of service to others.

Braving family opposition, Lillias first trained as a nurse at the Liverpool Workhouse Infirmary.[83] She followed this by studying medicine at the LSMW and in Edinburgh, graduating LRCP, in 1890 and completing her MD in Brussels.[84]

After graduating she travelled to Calcutta, India, and worked in a small private practice there in 1893 and 1894 and as physician-in-charge of the Lady Dufferin Hospital. Lillias contracted cholera in 1894 and went to Afghanistan to recuperate for a few months but remained in Kabul for three years as physician to the Court of the Amir, Abdur Rahman Khan.

In Kabul, Lillias' sister, who later trained in nursing, assisted Lillias when her house rapidly became a hospital. Every morning her garden would be full of people, especially women and children, waiting for the doctor's attention. Lillias documented her experiences in two books: *A Vizier's Daughter: A Tale of the Hazara War* (1900) and *A Nurse's Bequest* (1907), both published by John Murray in London. She was forced to return to England for surgery in 1897 and in London she developed a successful medical practice. She also travelled to South Africa, where she bought a farm in the Transvaal, later taken over by her brother Dundas.[85]

From 1908 to 1924 she was warden of Studley Horticultural and Agricultural College for Women at Studley Castle in Warwickshire and developed the school as one of the premier training colleges for women in England. Her period as warden was disrupted for a time when she volunteered for war work in 1915. Lillias was then aged fifty-seven but this did not stop her from joining the WARC and travelling to Montenegro, where she worked at a typhoid hospital beside Australian doctor Isabel Ormiston until the approach of the Austrian army forced their departure.

Post-war, Lillias returned to the college she had established. It was based on the concept that active outdoor work for women could be a health-giving career, and it provided training in a range of agricultural and horticultural jobs. Lillias felt strongly about the importance of constructive rather than destructive work and that working the land had healing possibilities. It was said that she had a forceful and brilliant personality and had an invigorating effect on the community of women.

In 1924 ill health forced her to retire from the college and she died in Nice, France, in early 1925, aged sixty-six.[86] A farmhand at the college said there was 'no-one like the doctor, if you were in real trouble; no-one like the doctor in appreciation of a joke, even against herself'.[87]

Dr Elizabeth Isabel Hamilton-Browne

1882–1985

Elizabeth Isabel Hamilton-Browne was born in 1882 in Sydney, the child of Henry Hamilton-Browne and Elizabeth Clark, and she was raised as a Quaker. Elizabeth was educated at Wellesley College in Newtown and was dux of her year when she matriculated in 1901. She began her medical degree at the University of Sydney in 1905 and won the Collie Prize for Botany and first class honours for biology in her first year.

Due to her excellent academic results, Elizabeth, along with Mary Boyd Williams, was one of the first women undergraduates appointed as prosectors[88] by the Faculty of Medicine. In her fifth year, 1909, Elizabeth was appointed a junior demonstrator, graduating MB, ChM, with first class honours, in 1910 – one of the first three women to achieve this. She then became the first woman to complete a residency in surgery at the Sydney Hospital in the same year. By 1915 she had been appointed as the hospital's pathologist and was also superintendent of the Royal Hospital for Women in Sydney.[89]

In late 1915 she sailed to England to participate in the war effort and in early 1916 was appointed as a surgeon to the Endell Street Military Hospital in London, with the ex-officio rank of captain. Following two years of surgical work she moved to the No. 19 General Hospital in Egypt and from early May 1918 was house surgeon at the Alexandria Hospital. Elizabeth completed her war work with a period in 1918 in France as a medical officer in charge of 500 American women clerks undertaking administration work for the British army.

Attracted to exotic places, in 1924 she went to Calcutta in West Bengal, India, to the Lady Dufferin Hospital where Dr Lillias Hamilton had worked thirty years before. In 1930 she was appointed vice-principal and professor of surgery at the Lady Hardinge Medical College for Women in Delhi and by 1939 she was in Lahore, India. During World War II she became assistant to the inspector-general of Civil Hospitals in the Punjab.

Her life of service was recognised by the British government in 1941 when she received the Member of the British Empire medal.[90] Elizabeth retired to Australia in 1952, to Hazelbrook in the Blue Mountains area of New South Wales, and died in 1985 at the age of 102.[91]

She is commemorated by the University of Sydney's Elizabeth and Henry Hamilton-Browne Scholarship to support medical research and to encourage female postgraduates in particular.

Dr Elaine Marjory Little

1884–1974

Elaine Marjory Little (known as Marjory) followed her Irish father's profession. He was Dr Joseph Henry Little, who married Agnes Elisabeth Mellor. After migrating to Australia, they had four daughters, and Marjory, the second, was born in 1884 in Brisbane. Marjory's mother died in 1890 when Marjory was just six years of age.[92] She attended school in Brisbane, then in England when her father took the family there between 1890 and 1900, and at the Girls' High School in Armidale, New South Wales, where her father set up practice on returning to Australia.

Distinctively tall in appearance, in 1906 she began studying science at the University of Sydney. After obtaining her BSc in 1911 she went on to study medicine and obtained her MB, ChM in 1915. At university her favourite subject was pathology and her expertise meant that she both tutored and demonstrated in the subject.

She began her pathology career as a junior resident medical officer at the Royal Prince Alfred Hospital in 1915 and became a senior resident in 1916–1917. In October 1917, Marjory became determined to serve in the war and her friend, the brilliant pathologist Dr Elsie Dalyell, already working in Malta, strongly encouraged her.

Marjory travelled independently to London, obtaining a position with the Lister Institute of Preventive Medicine. By this time, the RAMC was employing women doctors to serve and she was appointed an ex-officio captain in April 1918. Marjory was deployed to the 25th Stationary Hospital in Rouen, France, as a pathologist. While there, she wrote a research paper on 'Fatal Influenza Cases in British Army Hospitals in France' in collaboration with nurse and expert laboratory practitioner, Eleanor Williams.[93] Marjory worked at Rouen and at the Isolation Hospital at Étaples throughout 1918 and 1919 for the RAMC.

She sailed home to Sydney on the SS *Indarra* and returned to her work with Professor David Welsh at the University of Sydney in addition to setting up a very successful private pathology practice in the city. She was also consulting haematologist at Sydney Hospital and consulting pathologist for the Royal North Shore Hospital and the Rachel Forster Hospital for Women and Children. She found time to publish two articles about her war experiences in 1923.[94] In 1938 she became a Foundation Fellow of the Royal Australian College of Physicians and, in 1956, a Fellow of the Royal College of Pathologists of Australia.[95]

Marjory did not marry and settled at Pymble, New South Wales, with the youngest of her four sisters, Cicely, a teacher and novelist. She retired from her practice in 1952 and then had time to share Cicely's passion – the garden. In 1958 Marjory presented the postgraduate oration for the Medicine Faculty of the University of Sydney, paying tribute to her contemporaries and inspiring the younger medical women at the same time. She died in 1974, a month before her ninetieth birthday, at Lane Cove, Sydney.

Dr Mabel Murray-Prior

1882–1932

Mabel Murray-Prior was born into an outback Queensland family, at Bulli Bulli Station in western Queensland. Her father was Thomas Murray-Prior of Maroon Station in the Boonah district, a member of the Queensland parliament, and her mother was Florence Moore, from Bowen, north Queensland. Mabel had three sisters and a brother.

Mabel was sent to Sydney for her schooling at Ascham School at Edgecliff and matriculated to enter Sydney University.[96] She began studying an Arts degree in 1899, the forty-first woman student to enrol at the university, and she lived at the university's Women's College. After completing the first year of her Arts degree, she decided to study medicine and completed four years of the course in Sydney over a number of years. However, she did not finally complete her medical training until 1917 in Dublin.

In August 1914, Mabel was travelling and staying in Hong Kong. She left immediately for London when war was declared and volunteered to work as a hospital VAD throughout 1915. Observing that doctors were urgently needed, she resumed her medical studies in 1916, graduating in Dublin in 1917 and also completing her MD at the University of Edinburgh. Once qualified, Mabel was then appointed to the Royal Herbert Hospital in Greenwich for six months and then worked at Edinburgh Hospital till some months after the Armistice.[97]

In 1921 she returned to Australia for a visit and travelled for some years before settling down to country life in England and later in Ireland. She was described as 'a born sportswoman and took great pleasure in hunting and breeding dogs'.[98] These were her favourite pursuits from her early station life in Queensland. Mabel lived the final years of her life in Ireland, where she established a medical practice and took courses in gynaecology. In 1932 she suffered a severe fall and subsequently developed pneumonia, dying at the age of fifty. One of her friends described her as 'a lady of brilliant intellect and vivid personality and had a good practice and a large circle of friends'.[99]

Dr Martha Isabel Ormiston (Garvice)

1883–1958

In 1880, Andrew and Sarah Ormiston and their children migrated to Australia from Bailieborough in County Cavan, Ireland, to live in Newton, a small town south of Albury, New South Wales. Andrew's brother Joseph had made the same trip in 1860 and his cartage business was prospering. Although the family had lived in Ireland, the Ormiston name and origins are Scottish. It is likely that during the previous two centuries, some part of the family had left Scotland and settled in Bailieborough, on the estate of William Bailie of Aye, a fellow Scot.

Martha Isabel (known as Isabel) was born three years later; she was one of nine children, four boys and five girls. The younger Ormiston family members, including Isabel, were educated at the small Albury Superior Public School, later called Riverina Grammar. In her final school year, Isabel won the Classics prize and then enrolled in Arts at the University of Sydney in 1901. However, medicine seemed more appealing to her and the following year she began the five-year degree in medicine and surgery as one of the medical faculty's early female students. When she began her first year in 1902, only eleven women had previously graduated in medicine from the University of Sydney.

Isabel was also a boarder at the pioneering Women's College, opened in 1894, the first residential community of female under-graduates to be established in Australian universities. At the college, Isabel became part of a small community of twenty-five women students, one of whom was fellow medical student Eleanor Bourne, who would also serve in World War I.[100]

Isabel's four brothers all became pharmacists and dentists and one of her four sisters, Sarah, trained as a nurse. When Isabel graduated, permanent hospital appointments and other medical positions were exceptionally difficult for women to obtain. She completed her residency at the Bowen Hospital for Children in Brisbane but then, like many early female graduates in Great Britain and Australia, her career began in the public health sector when she took up the position of health inspector of Tasmanian schools in September 1910.[101]

Although positions in public health were not viewed as professional prizes by the male medical fraternity, they provided young female graduates with financial security, independence from family and unchaperoned mobility. In her new role, Isabel travelled constantly around Tasmania and was invited to the social events that were written up in the daily newspapers. She favoured outfits in pale blue, and hats trimmed with ostrich feathers.

In mid-1914 she took leave to travel to London to attend the Victoria League Conference on Child Health with the intention also of completing a Diploma of Public Health, a course for medical inspectors at the University of Edinburgh.[102] Edinburgh's medical school was a world leader at the time in the developing area of public health and at least five Australian and New Zealand women doctors who served during World War I completed their medical training there.

Isabel was in Ireland when she heard that war had broken out, and she initially joined the Red Cross in London and then went to the WARC, serving at their hospital at Ostend on the Belgian coast in 1914 and being taken prisoner of war when the German army invaded. She returned to work at the L'Hôpital de L'Ocean, the Queen of the Belgians' Hospital in La Panne in early 1915.

The WARC then posted Isabel to work at their hospital in Montenegro until she was forced to retreat ahead of the Austrian army, undertaking a perilous eight-day trip, often on horseback, through the Dinaric Alps to reach Salonica. She worked for the British Red Cross Convalescent Depot, Egypt, in 1916. In 1917 the WARC sent her to their hospital in Limoges, France, where she served until April 1918. Isabel was mentioned in dispatches for gallant action in the face of the enemy in Ostend, Belgium, as well as receiving the Montenegrin Red Cross and the Order of Danilo for her work in Montenegro.

In 1919 Isabel obtained a position in Egypt as a schools medical inspector.[103] The following year, in January 1920, she married Major Chudleigh Garvice, who was Commandant of the Alexandria Police in Egypt. He died unexpectedly fourteen months later and they had no children. Isabel remained with the Egyptian Ministry of Education in Alexandria, as the Senior Lady Medical Officer, where in 1928 she was made a MBE for her services to the community.

In 1935 it was reported that, as the Senior Lady Medical Officer, Isabel had a staff of five English women doctors and forty Egyptian nurses caring for the health of over 40,000 school children. Much of the work centred around the prevention and treatment of eyesight problems.

A tiny woman, weighing only fifty kilograms, Isabel remained adventurous into her later years. In 1935 she was the first woman passenger to travel by Imperial Airways from Egypt to Australia. It was Isabel's first flight and the journey to Australia took eleven days, flying over Egypt, Persia and India. It enabled her to visit her family in Australia, rather than spending her two months of annual leave in England.[104]

During World War II, Isabel stayed at her work in Egypt and additionally acted as anaesthetist in one of Cairo's military hospitals. She was awarded an OBE for her services. After retiring in

1949, Isabel returned to Australia and her family in Sydney and died in Vaucluse in July 1958.

Dr Vera Scantlebury (Brown)

1889–1946

Vera Scantlebury was tiny when she was born on 7 August 1889 and her twin brother, George, did not survive more than a few hours. She was born in the gold-mining town of Linton in Victoria to Catherine Millington Baynes, the local postmistress, and Dr George Scantlebury.[105] The family moved to their newly built house, called Marathon, in the Melbourne bayside suburb of Cheltenham shortly after and grew to include Vera's brother Cliff and two sisters, Dorothy and Eileen. From a genteel but poor family of thirteen, Vera's mother, Catherine, had had to make her living before her marriage with only a meagre education and was resolute that all of her children would receive an education that would provide financial independence.

Vera was educated at Toorak College and the University of Melbourne medical school, and boarded at the Janet Clark Hostel, where a sign on her door read 'Scant-"ll"-bury while you wait'. Vera graduated MB, BS, in early 1914 and spent a year as a resident at the Melbourne Hospital, followed by residency at Melbourne's Children's Hospital. By the end of 1916 she had become the first woman to reach the position of senior resident at the Children's Hospital.

In February 1917 Vera departed her treasured position at the Children's Hospital to serve as a surgeon at the extraordinary 560-bed Endell Street Military Hospital in London, which was the creation of suffragettes Dr Louisa Garrett Anderson and

Dr Flora Murray. Vera served with the ex-officio rank of lieutenant for almost two years, returning to Melbourne in February
1919.[106]

Vera had revelled in her work at the Children's Hospital
before leaving for London and her intention on returning was to
develop a practice in the burgeoning specialty of paediatrics. In
1919 she accepted a part-time position as medical officer for the
Victorian Baby Health Centres Association and in 1924 took a
whirlwind trip through Canada and America to study child health
with leading practitioners and complete her MD. For six years she
applied for honorary positions at the Children's Hospital, the first
and very necessary step to becoming a paediatrician, but she was
continually passed over in favour of younger and less experienced
male applicants. Preference for returned servicemen, combined
with attitudes to women doctors that were essentially unchanged
by the war, meant that access to hospital positions was severely
limited.

In 1925, desperately disappointed by another unsuccessful
application, Vera gave up. But in the same year she presented extensive and informed evidence to the Commonwealth government's
Royal Commission on Health and was asked by the Victorian
government in 1926 to conduct an enquiry into the health of
women and children of Victoria, along with Dr Henrietta Main.[107]

Late in 1926, the Victorian government established the
Department of Infant Welfare within the Department of Public
Health and Vera was appointed as the pioneer Director – the first
woman to head a government department in Victoria. In the same
month she married Dr Edward Byam Brown and her appointment
was rapidly made part-time.

Between 1926 and 1946, Vera developed a professional, state-
wide infant welfare system that remains the basis of maternal

and child health in Victoria today. Vera and Eddie had two children – Edward in 1928 and Catherine in 1931 – and Vera's achievement in developing a state-wide policy and system while being a working mother was an exceptional one. She was awarded an OBE in 1938 in recognition of her contribution to infant health in both Victoria and the Commonwealth of Australia.

Vera died at the age of fifty-six in 1946, and her achievements are commemorated annually with the awarding of the Dr Vera Scantlebury Brown Memorial Trust Scholarship and biennially with the Dr Vera Scantlebury Brown Oration at the University of Melbourne.[108]

Dr Hannah Mary Helen Sexton

1862–1950

Hannah Mary Helen Sexton (known as Helen) played a seminal role in the history of Victoria. In 1887 she and Lilian Alexander challenged contemporary female gender restrictions when they approached the Melbourne University Council for permission to become the first women to enrol in medicine in the state. They advertised in *The Argus* for other interested women to join them, which created a great deal of public interest. Subsequently, Helen Sexton was one of the first seven women to enrol in the Melbourne University medical school in late 1887, beginning her studies in 1888. Graduating MB, BS in 1892, she was the third woman to do so in Victoria.

Helen Sexton, born 21 June 1862, was the fifth and youngest child of Maria Bromwell and Daniel Sexton, an Irish migrant architect and builder. She attended Carlton Ladies' College and, after matriculating, enrolled in an Arts degree at the University of

Melbourne in the early 1880s. As her mother was against Helen's
dream of becoming a doctor, Helen waited until after her mother's
death to begin her campaign to allow women into the medical
faculty and, finally, to enrol in medicine.[109]

In 1896, Helen Sexton was among the six women doctors,
led by Dr Constance Stone, to found the first women's hospital
in Melbourne – the Queen Victoria Hospital for Women and
Children. It began its life in a hall at the rear of the Welsh
Church in La Trobe Street, where medicines were dispensed
and poor women could receive free treatment. The doctor's
room, ward and dispensary window remain in existence at the
church today.

Three years later Helen Sexton was elected as the first woman
honorary gynaecological surgeon to the Women's Hospital,
Melbourne, the first at any Melbourne hospital.[110] She proved to
be a very skilful surgeon, was popular and had a good sense of
humour, working harmoniously with the male surgeons at the
hospital. Health problems forced her to retire early from her position at the Women's in 1910, and she sailed to London in 1912,
travelling around Europe until 1914.

At the age of fifty-two, and still in Europe, she offered her
services to the RAMC in London soon after the declaration of
war but was rejected. Determined to assist in the war, she changed
course and returned home to Melbourne to raise money for her
own military hospital in France. Other Australian women joined
her venture and she opened the Hôpital Australien de Paris at
Auteuil in July 1915. Later that year she took up a surgical position
at the Val de Grâce Military Hospital nearby.

In 1917 Helen Sexton returned to Melbourne, resuming her
practice and settling in Toorak. She was well known in society,
wearing hats and 'sensible shoes'; she was charming and had

a 'broad sense of humour'. It was said that Helen was 'terribly serious about . . . life and duty, but she had a love of fun as well'.[111]

Never marrying, two years later in 1919 she retired and again travelled to Europe, living in Florence, Italy, where she worked among the poor for almost thirty years, despite suffering from severe arthritis. She died in London on 12 October 1950.[112] Of the group of women doctors who founded the Queen Victoria Hospital in St David's Church Hall on La Trobe Street in 1896, Helen reflected:

> In that band there were no self-seekers. We knew and felt how great the need for such a hospital would be, so body, brain and spirit were put into our efforts, and it was one great and splendid pull together, and the joy was as great as the work.[113]

Dr Isabella Henrietta Younger (Ross)

1887–1956

Isabella Henrietta Younger was brought up in the south-western Victorian coastal town of Warrnambool, the eldest of four daughters born to Henrietta and her husband, John Younger, an Irishman who had migrated to Australia via Canada. John Younger had become a prominent member of the Warrnambool community, opening Younger's Department Store in the main street and holding the office of Mayor in 1912–1913.

Isabella earned a gold medal as dux of her secondary school, Warrnambool's Hohenlohe Ladies' College. Uncommonly for a girls' school, the college offered matriculation subjects for entry to university. Isabella began her medical degree at the University of Melbourne but travelled to Glasgow to complete the final year in 1914. She then decided to expand her experience by working for a time in the poverty-stricken slum areas of Edinburgh and Glasgow.[114]

She moved to London later in 1915 when she was appointed as house physician to the Queen's Hospital for Children in Bethnal Green in London. At Queen's she worked with Dr Eric Pritchard, who was an early expert in the nascent areas of child and maternal health and the development of infant welfare centres.[115]

While in London she met Melbourne merchant John Ross and they married in April 1916. During that year Isabella contributed to the war effort by helping at London's Waterloo Station when convoys of wounded arrived and by working for a time at a military hospital in Kent. Later that year she and John journeyed home through America and Isabella took the opportunity to look at the work of Dr Herman Bundesen of Chicago, another early proponent of the importance of reducing the rates of infant mortality amid the poor living conditions of industrial cities.

Both Pritchard and Bundesen inspired Isabella to consider what could be done when she returned to Melbourne in 1917 and found that infant mortality in the city's inner industrial suburbs was between ten and fifteen per cent. She gathered a group of concerned and determined women around her because 'We were tired of trying to convince everyone we met that the only way to reduce the terrible havoc of suffering and sickness amongst babies was by prevention – keeping the well-baby well' and together they opened Victoria's first baby health centre in Richmond.[116]

Within five years they had created the Victorian Baby Health Centres Association (VBHCA), acquired council funding, set up a training centre for infant welfare nurses, appointed two outstanding women – Dr Vera Scantlebury as medical officer and Sister Muriel Peck as head of the training school – and established thirty-eight city and six country centres. All the VBHCA organisational and fundraising work was done voluntarily and heavily influenced by the enthusiastic leadership of Isabella.[117]

Isabella worked voluntarily for the VBHCA for more than thirty years and founded a system of maternal and child health which became the universal service that still exists in Victoria today. Her only child, a son, was killed on active service in New Guinea during World War II. Isabella died in 1956, her name commemorated at Warrnambool's Isabella Younger Ross Maternal and Child Health Centre in Fairy Street.

Notes and references

Introduction

1   *The Common Cause*, vol. VII, no. 333, 27 August 1915, p. 1
2   Murray, Flora, *Women as Army Surgeons*, Hodder & Stoughton, London, c. 1920, p. 4
3   Sinclair, May, *A Journal of Impressions in Belgium*, The Macmillan Company, New York, 1915, p. 69
4   Scantlebury Brown, Vera, Diary letters, University of Melbourne Archive, 1984.0082, 1917–1939, vol. A14, October 1918, p. 10

Chapter 1: 'The War Office regrets'

1   *Sydney Morning Herald*, 10 May 1915, p. 8
2   Lee, Ruth L., *Woman War Doctor: The Life of Mary De Garis*, Australian Scholarly Publishing, Melbourne, 2014, p. 65
3   *Sydney Morning Herald*, 12 November 1914, p. 9
4   Nairn, Bede, 'Forster, William (1818–1882)', *Australian Dictionary of Biography*, National Centre of Biography, Australian National University, http://adb.anu.edu.au/biography/forster-william
5   Clark, Matilda Emily, *A War Nurse's Diary: Sketches from a Belgian War Hospital*, The Macmillan Company, New York, 1918, p. 8
6   Souttar, Henry Sessions, *A Surgeon in Belgium*, Edward Arnold, London, 1915, p. 4
7   Lazovic, Ivana & Sujic, Radmila, 'Women Doctors in the Serbian Sanitary Service during the Balkan Wars', *Acta Medico-historica Adriatica*, vol. 5, no. 1, 2007, pp. 71–82
8   *The Common Cause*, vol. VIII, no. 412, 2 March 1917, pp. 625–6
9   Clark, *A War Nurse's Diary*, p. 8
10 Souttar, *A Surgeon in Belgium*, pp. 8–9
11 Hallam, Andrew & Hallam, Nicola (eds), *Lady under Fire on the Western Front: The Great War Letters of Lady Dorothie Feilding MM*, Pen & Sword Books, Yorkshire, 2011, pp. 8–11

12 Clark, *A War Nurse's Diary*, p. 9
13 'The Millicent Fawcett Hospital Units', *The Common Cause*, vol. VIII, no. 412, 2 March 1917, pp. 625–6
14 Gatrell, Peter & Zvanko, Liubov (eds), *Europe on the Move: Refugees in the Era of the Great War*, Oxford University Press, Oxford, 2017, p. 11
15 *Newcastle Journal*, 28 September 1914, p. 5; *Jus Suffragii*, 1 November 1915, vol. 10, no. 2, p. 25
16 *Singleton Argus*, 13 April 1916, p. 4
17 Clark, *A War Nurse's Diary*, pp. 21–2
18 'The Millicent Fawcett Hospital Units', *The Common Cause*, pp. 625–6
19 'Women Under Fire', *The British Journal of Nursing*, 17 October 1914, p. 305
20 Souttar, *A Surgeon in Belgium*, p. 90
21 Sinclair, *A Journal of Impressions in Belgium*, pp. 268, 271
22 Ramsay, Mabel L., *Women's Imperial Service Hospital at Antwerp, Notes and Diary of Events from 16 September to 14 October 1914*, www.scarletfinders.co.uk/165.html
23 Sinclair, *A Journal of Impressions in Belgium*, p. 276
24 *Hawera & Normanby Star*, 13 May 1915
25 *The Sun* (Sydney), 2 May 1915, p. 16
26 'British Expelled from Ostend', *Evening Telegraph*, 26 October 1914, p. 3
27 *The Sun* (Sydney), 2 May 1915, p. 16
28 Hallett, Christine E, *Veiled Warriors: Allied Nurses of the First World War*, Oxford University Press, Oxford, 2014, pp. 40–1
29 *Jus Suffragii*, 1 November 1915, vol. 10, no. 2, p. 25
30 *The Sun* (Sydney), 2 May 1915, p. 16
31 It is not possible to be certain of Dr Laura Forster's return to Belgium with the BFH. This statement is based on the comparison of a photograph of Laura in a Sydney newspaper with the photo of the surgical team at Furnes and on Matilda Emily Clark's diary entry that the only remaining female doctor was undertaking this role.

Chapter 2: 'Beyond description'

1 'An Australian in Servia'[sic], *Sydney Morning Herald*, 30 June 1915, p. 5
2 Krippner, Monica, *The Quality of Mercy: Women at War, 1915–1918*, David & Charles, London, 1980, pp. 34–35

3   Wright, James R Jr & Baskin, Leland B, 'Pathology and Laboratory Medicine Support for the American Expeditionary Forces by the US Army Medical Corps during World War I', *Archives of Pathology & Laboratory Medicine*, September 2015, vol. 139, no. 9, pp. 1161–72

4   Tschanz, David W, 'Typhus Fever on the Eastern Front in World War I', www.entomology.montana/edu/historybug/wwi

5   'An Australian in Servia'[sic], *Sydney Morning Herald*, 30 June 1915, p. 5

6   *The Common Cause*, 7 January 1916, p. 522

7   'Extracts from a Serbian Letter by Dr Dalyell', *The Magazine of the Women's College*, November 1915, pp. 37–41

8   Ibid.

9   'With the Serbians', *Nelson Evening Mail*, vol. XLIX, 12 November 1915, p. 2

10   Letter from Elsie Dalyell to Professor David Welsh, University of Sydney, http://beyond1914.sydney.edu.au/profile/2736/elsie-jean-dalyell

11   Ibid.

12   Letter from Professor David Welsh to University of Sydney archives, 21 October 1915, http://beyond1914.sydney.edu.au/profile/2736/elsie-jean-dalyell

13   Maitland, T Gwynne, 'Notes on the Typhus Epidemic in Serbia', *British Medical Journal*, 21 August 1915, p. 283

14   'Extracts from a Serbian letter by Dr Dalyell', *The Magazine of the Women's College*, November 1915, pp. 37–41

15   Ibid.

16   Application for Admission, Student's Form, London (Royal Free Hospital) School for Women, Women's College archives, University of Sydney

17   Geddes, Jennian, 'Women as Army Surgeons: The Women's Hospital Corps', MA thesis, London Metropolitan University, May 2005, p. 18

18   *Lost Hospitals of London*, http://ezitis.myzen.co.uk/kinggeorge stamford.html

19   *The Lancet*, vol. 185, 26 June 1915, p. 1376

20   *West Australian*, 23 April 1915, p. 7

21   Miles, Hallie Eustace, *Untold Tales of War-Time London: A Personal Diary*, Cecil Palmer, London, 1930, p. 41. Hallie Miles visited Victoria Station on 5 March 1915

22 *British Journal of Nursing*, 15 May 1915, p. 417

23 *The Mercury*, 20 November 1915, p. 5

24 Stebbing, EP, *At the Serbian Front in Macedonia*, John Lane, London, 1917, p. 32

25 *British Journal of Nursing*, 12 June 1915, p. 507

26 Hoyle, Gwyneth, *Flowers in the Snow*, University of Nebraska Press, Lincoln, 2001, p. 25

27 *The Mercury*, 20 November 1915, p. 5

28 Possibly Mt Bjeshket e Nemuna, but this cannot be confirmed.

29 McQuellen, Christopher, 'Doctor Isabel Ormiston', *Albury & District Historical Society Bulletin*, vol. 541, p. 5

30 Manson, Cecil & Manson, Celia, *Dr Agnes Bennett*, Michael Joseph, London, 1960, p. 24

31 Manson & Manson, *Dr Agnes Bennett*, p. 71

32 *Daily Herald*, 22 April 1915, p. 4

33 Trinca, John C, 'Kitchener's Hundred', *Chiron*, vol. 2, no. 4, p. 57

34 Plowman, Peter, *Across the Sea to War: Australian and New Zealand Troopships from 1865*, Rosenberg Publishing, Sydney, 2003, p. 64

35 *Treating Gallipoli's Wounded–Dr Agnes Bennett*, http://anzacsight sound.org/audios/treating-gallipoli-s-wounded-dr-agnes-bennett

36 Manson & Manson, *Dr Agnes Bennett*, p. 72

37 Maclean, Hester, *Nursing in New Zealand: History and Reminiscences*, Tolan Printing Company, 1932, p. 162

38 Bowerbank, Major, *New Zealand Hospitals in Egypt: The War Effort of New Zealand*, Whitcomb & Tombs, Auckland, 1923, p. 114

39 Barrett, JW & Dean, PE, *The AAMC in Egypt*, HK Lewis, London, 1918, p. 54

40 Manson & Manson, *Dr Agnes Bennett*, p. 73

41 *Kai Teaki*, vol. IX, no. 2, April 1916, p. 86

42 The Lister Institute, 'Our History: The Early Years', www.lister-institute.org.uk/about-us/our-history/

43 Letter from Emma Buckley to Sir Thomas Anderson Stuart, 28 July, 1915, http://beyond1914.sydney.edu.au/profile/2552/emma-albani-buckley-turkington

44 The Lister Institute, 'Our History: Contributing During Two World Wars', www.lister-institute.org.uk/about-us/our-history/

45 Cox, Francis, 'The First World War: Disease, the Only Victor', www.gresham.ac.uk/lectures-and-events/the-first-world-war-disease-the-only-victor

46   Geddes, Jennian, 'Deeds not Words in the Suffrage Military
     Hospital in Endell Street', *Medical History*, vol. 51, no. 1, 2007,
     p. 79
47   Geddes, 'Women as Army Surgeons', pp. 24–5
48   Murray, Flora, *Women as Army Surgeons*, 2nd edition, Cambridge
     University Press, London, 2014, p. 5
49   Geddes, 'Women as Army Surgeons', pp. 25–7
50   Murray, *Women as Army Surgeons*, p. 99
51   Geddes, 'Women as Army Surgeons', p. 43
52   Murray, *Women as Army Surgeons*, p. 102
53   Letter from Emma Buckley to Sir Thomas Anderson Stuart,
     5 February 1918, p. 2, http://beyond1914.sydney.edu.au/profile/
     2552/emma-albani-buckley-turkington
54   'Australian Hospital Opened in France', *The Argus*, 6 August 1915,
     p. 8
55   Dease, Arthur, 'World War I Letters Home from the Western
     Front', 8 July 1915 and 4 September 1915, www.arthursletters.com/
     ww1-letters-home.html; 'Notes and News', *The Common Cause*,
     vol. 7, no. 333, 27 August 1915, p. 1
56   Helen Sexton Casebook, Manuscript 2189, Australian Medical
     Association Archive, University of Melbourne Medical History
     Museum
57   'Vice-Regal', *The Argus*, 20 November 1919, p. 6
58   *Sydney Morning Herald*, 27 May 1937, p. 20
59   *The Mirror of Australia*, 13 November 1915, p. 17
60   *Glenn Innes Examiner*, 8 November 1915, p. 5
61   *Richmond River Herald*, 16 November 1915, p. 3
62   Queen Alexandra's Royal Army Nursing Corps, 'Voluntary Aid
     Detachment', www.qaranc.co.uk/voluntary-aid-detachment.php;
     Cohen, Susan, *Medical Services in the First World War*, Shire
     Publications, Oxford, 2014, pp. 5–6, 11
63   Lee, Ruth L, *Woman War Doctor: The Life of Mary De Garis*,
     Australian Scholarly Publishing, Melbourne, 2014, p. 79
64   In an area of contested sovereignty and borders, we have adopted
     the place name used by the SWH for their Ostrovo hospital at the
     time, i.e. SWH America Unit in Macedonia with the Serbian army.
65   Lee, *Woman War Doctor*, p. 79
66   'Millicent Fawcett Hospital Units for Refugees in Russia', *British
     Journal of Nursing*, 20 January 1917, p. 50

67 Edwards, Nina, *Dressed for War: Uniform, Civilian Clothing & Trappings, 1914–1918*, L. B. Tauris & Co, London, 2014, pp. 4–8

68 Letter from Laura Fowler Hope (Wootton Sea, UK) to George Swan Fowler (Adelaide), 21 May 1898. Despite the fact that few written sources by Laura Fowler Hope about her war years have survived, crucially her war diary and some letters have been kept. The Fowler Family Papers, number PRG34, are in the Mortlock Library of South Australia, State Library of South Australia, Adelaide.

69 Secomb, Robin, 'Borne in Empire: Issues of Gender, Ethnicity and Power behind Laura Fowler Hope's Journey to Kalimpong', *Outskirts Online Journal*, vol. 7, November 2000, www.outskirts.arts. uwa.edu.au/volumes/volume-7/secomb/

70 Ibid.

71 Laura Fowler Hope, Diary 1915–1916, p. 1

72 Leneman, Leah, *In the Service of Life, the Story of Elsie Inglis and the Scottish Women's Hospitals*, Mercat Press, Edinburgh, 1994, p. 25.

73 Ibid., p. 39.

74 Ibid., p. 28.

75 Laura Fowler Hope, Diary 1915–1916, pp. 2–8

76 Ibid., p. 5

77 Johnston, Olive (ed), *The Hands of a Woman*, Wakefield Press, Adelaide, 1994, p. 33

78 Laura Fowler Hope, Diary 1915–1916, p. 13

79 'Prisoners in Austria', *Queensland Figaro*, 22 April 1916, p. 11.

80 Alice Hutchinson in Leneman, *In the Service of Life*, p. 44.

81 Ibid.

82 'Prisoners in Austria', *Queensland Figaro*, 22 April 1916, p. 11.

83 Laura Fowler Hope, Diary 1915–1916, p. 19.

84 Leneman, *In the Service of Life*, p. 44.

85 Ibid., p. 45.

86 Laura Fowler Hope, Diary 1915–1916, p. 28

87 Krippner, *The Quality of Mercy*, p. 162

88 Leneman, *In the Service of Life*, p. 50

89 Laura Fowler Hope, Diary 1915–1916, p. 29

90 Jones, Helen, 'Hope, Laura Margaret (1868–1952)', *Australian Dictionary of Biography*, vol. 14, Melbourne University Press, 1996, p. 491

91 Bassett, Jan, *Guns and Brooches: Australian Army Nursing from the Boer War to the Gulf War*, Oxford University Press, Melbourne, 1992, p. 36

92 *National Advocate*, 8 February 1916, p. 4

93 Tudor, Spencer (ed), *World War I: Encyclopedia Vol 1*, ABC-CLIO, Santa Barbara, 2005, p. 118

94 *British Journal of Nursing*, 5 February 1916, p. 117; and 29 April 1916, p. 376

95 King-Hall, Stephen, *North Sea Diary, 1914–1918*, Newnes, London, 1936, www.vlib.us/wwi/resources/northseadiary.html#no9

96 *British Journal of Nursing*, 6 November 1915, p. 377

97 *The Common Cause*, 4 February 1916, p. 570

98 Galicia no longer exists as a nation-state. World War I-era Galicia would today straddle the borders of Poland and the Ukraine, but mostly be situated in western Ukraine.

99 Storr, Katherine, *Excluded from the Record: Women, Refugees and Relief, 1914–1929*, Peter Lang, Bern, 2010, pp. 229–30

100 Mellor, Lise, *150 Years, 150 Firsts: The People of the Faculty of Medicine*, Sydney University Press, 2006, p. 14

101 Letter from Elizabeth Hamilton-Browne to Sir Thomas Anderson Stuart, 21 February 1916, http://beyond1914.sydney.edu.au/profile/3084/elizabeth-isabel-leila-hamilton-browne

Chapter 3: 'The bullets were singing all over the field'

1 Creswick, P, Pond, G & Ashton, P, *Kent's Care for the Wounded*, Hodder & Stoughton, London, 1915, pp. 55–6

2 Eleanor Elizabeth Bourne Papers, State Library of Queensland, SLQ OM81-130, unpublished manuscript, 'Twenty Eight Years Ago', p. 1

3 Williams, Lesley M, *No Better Profession: Medical Women in Queensland, 1891–1999*, Watson, Ferguson & Co, Brisbane, 2006, pp. 13–14

4 Bourne, 'Twenty Eight Years Ago', p. 1

5 Geddes, 'Women as Army Surgeons', pp. 136–7

6 Scantlebury Brown, Vera, Diary letters, vol. A3, June 1917, p. 68

7 Bourne, 'Twenty Eight Years Ago', p. 2

8 Bourne, 'Twenty Eight Years Ago', p. 6

9 Officer, Doris, *An Appreciation*, Baby Health, Victorian Baby Health Centres Association, c. April 1956

10 'British Red Cross Transport during the First World War', www.redcross.org.uk/volunteers-during-WWI

11 *Warrnambool Standard*, 24 June 1916, p. 5

12 Creswick, Pond & Ashton, *Kent's Care for the Wounded*, pp. 55–6

13 1st AIF Personnel Records 1914–1920, Series B2455, 'Archibald

Darling Gould', www.naa.gov.au/collection/explore/defence/service-records/

14 Family notes and memories provided by Richard Shaw, Rachel's third child

15 Barwick, Archie, *In Great Spirits: Archie Barwick's WWI Diary*, HarperCollins, Sydney, 2013, Kindle Edition

16 *Sydney Morning Herald*, 3 November 1916, p. 6

17 Clayton, Anthony, *Paths of Glory: The French Army 1914–1918*, Cassell, London, 2003, p. 110

18 *Townsville Daily Bulletin*, 24 November 1916, p. 6

19 Ibid.

20 Manson & Manson, *Dr Agnes Bennett*, p. 75

21 Manson & Manson, *Dr Agnes Bennett*, p. 7

Chapter 4: 'At the bottom of a deep narrow shell wound'

1 Elsie Dalyell in Crofton, Eileen, *The Women of Royaumont: A Scottish Women's Hospital on the Western Front*, Tuckwell Press, East Lothian, 1997, p. 75

2 Powell, Anne, *Women in the War Zone: Hospital Service in the First World War*, The History Press, Gloucestershire, 2009, pp. 25, 161

3 'The Women's Hospital', *Auckland Star*, 16 May 1917, p. 7

4 Leneman, *In the Service of Life*, p. 55

5 The French name for the hospital was Hôpital Auxiliare 301

6 Holmes, Grace, 'Frances Ivens, MB, MS Lond, ChM Liverp.', http://www.kumc.edu/wwi/essays-on-first-world-war-medicine/index-of-essays/biography/frances-ivens.html

7 Crofton, *The Women of Royaumont*, pp. 19–20

8 Sister Leila Smith (Australian nurse) in Butler, AG, *Official History of the Australian Army Medical Corps*, Australian War Memorial, Melbourne, 1943, p. 408

9 *The Medical Journal of Australia*, vol. 11, no. 11, 13 September 1968, p. 349

10 Dalyell, EJ, 'A Case of Gangrene Associated with B. Oedematics', *British Medical Journal*, 17 March, 1917, p. 361

11 Crofton, *The Women of Royaumont*, p. 74

12 *Liverpool Daily Post*, 7 August 1916

13 Weiner, MF, 'The Scottish Women's Hospital at Royaumont, France 1914–1919', *Journal of the Royal College of Physicians of Edinburgh*, vol. 44, 2014, p. 329

14   Letter by Vera Collum, a Royaumont orderly, published in *The Great War*, vol. V, no. 71, 25 December 1915, p. 190

15   Crofton, *The Women of Royaumont*, p. 269

16   McQuellin, Christopher, 'Dr Isabel Ormiston', *Albury & District Historical Society Bulletin*, no. 541, December 2013, p. 5

17   Murray, *Women as Army Surgeons*, p. 99

18   Ibid., p. 3

19   'Malta RAMC: Military Hospitals Malta during the Great War 1914–1918', http://maltaramc.com/articles/contents/greatwar.html

20   Bowen, Claire, 'WAACs: Crossing the Line in the Great War', *Miranda*, vol. 2, 2010, pp. 2–8

21   The process for becoming an officer in the British army required the appointment to be officially gazetted.

22   Smythe, Percy, 'The World War I Diary of Percy Smythe', www.smythe.id.au/diary/ch3.htm

23   Brittain, Vera, *War Diary 1913–1917*, Alan Bishop (ed), Gollancz, 1981, p. 112

24   Bruce, GR, 'Malta Military Hospitals 1915–1917: Military Hospitals in Malta during the War, A Short Account of Their Inception and Development', www.scarletfinders.co.uk/190.html

25   Leneman, *In the Service of Life*, p. 71.

26   'The Women's Hospital', *Auckland Star*, 16 May 1917, p. 7

27   Leneman, *In the Service of Life*, p. 71

28   'The Women's Hospital', *Auckland Star*, 16 May 1917, p. 7

29   Krippner, *The Quality of Mercy*, p. 189

30   Lilian Cooper in Williams, Lesley M., *No Easy Path: The Life and Times of Lilian Violet Cooper*, Department of Child Health Publishing Unit, Royal Children's Hospital, Brisbane, 1991, p. 51

31   Manson & Manson, *Doctor Agnes Bennett*, p. 88

32   Agnes Bennett, 1914 Diary, Agnes Elizabeth Lloyd Bennett, 1872–1960, MS-Papers-1346, National Library of New Zealand, Wellington, NZ. 'Wad' is the gun cartridge that holds the shot together.

33   Williams, *No Easy Path*, p. 51

34   Ibid., p. 11

35   Ibid., p. 21; Cramond, Tess, 'Lilian Violet Cooper, MD, FRACS, Royal Australasian College of Surgeons', *Australia New Zealand Journal of Surgery*, no. 63, 1993, p. 106

36   Leneman, *In the Service of Life*, p. 86

37 Bennett, Agnes, 'With Our Allies in the Balkans: Work of the Women's Hospital Units' (lecture), *Dominion*, vol. 11, no. 137, 27 February 1918, p. 3

38 'Account of America Unit' (manuscript), Scottish Women's Hospitals, Imperial War Museum, London, BRCS. 24.4/58

39 Manson & Manson, *Doctor Agnes Bennett*, p. 92

40 Ibid., p. 103

41 Bennett, Agnes, 'With the Serbians', *Sydney Morning Herald*, 26 December 1917, p. 6

42 Leneman, *In the Service of Life*, p. 88

43 Letter from Agnes Bennett, Ostrovo, to Mrs Russell, Edinburgh, 20 July 1917, SWH Archive, Mitchell Library, Glasgow

44 Bennett, 'With the Serbians', *Sydney Morning Herald*, p. 6

45 Agnes Elizabeth Lloyd Bennett, 1872–1960, MS-Papers-1346, Alexander Turnbull Library, National Library of New Zealand

46 De Garis, MC, *Clinical Notes and Deductions of a Peripatetic: Being Fads and Fancies of a General Practitioner*, Bailliere, Tindall and Cox, London, 1926, p. 159

47 De Garis, *Clinical Notes and Deductions*, p. 67

48 Marlow, Joyce (ed), *The Virago Book of Women in the Great War*, Virago, London, 2011, p. 238

49 Ibid., p. 63

50 'Queensland Lady Doctor: Good Work in Serbia', *The Queenslander* (Brisbane), 21 April 1917, p. 5

51 Williams, *No Easy Path*, p. 59

52 The four major hospital ships fitted to carry thousands of wounded were the *Olympic*, the *Mauretania*, the *Aquitania* and the *Britannic*.

53 Brittain, Vera, *Testament of Youth*, Wideview Books, USA, 1980, pp. 297–98

54 Ibid., p. 300

55 Smythe, 'The World War I Diary of Percy Smythe', www.smythe.id.au/diary/Ch3.htm

56 Bruce, 'Military Hospitals in Malta', www.scarletfinders.co.uk/190.html

57 Walsh, Michael, *Brothers in War*, Random House, London, 2011, p. 313

58 Lost Hospitals of London, 'King George Hospital', http://ezitis.myzen.co.uk/kinggeorgestamford.html

59 Letter from Emma Buckley to Sir Thomas Anderson Stuart, 5 February 1918, http://beyond1914.sydney.edu.au/

60 Gammage, Bill, *The Broken Years: Australian Soldiers in the Great War*, Australian National University Press, Canberra, 1974, pp. 205–6; Woollacott, Angela, *Gender and Empire*, Palgrave Macmillan, London, 2006, pp. 129–132

61 Winter, Jay & Robert, Jean-Louis, *Capital Cities at War: Paris, London, Berlin 1914–1919*, Cambridge University Press, New York, 2007, p. 28; *Official Yearbook of the Commonwealth of Australia*, No. 11, Commonwealth Government, 1918, p. 124

62 Bassett, *Guns and Brooches*, p. 66

63 Scantlebury Brown, Vera, Diary letters, vol. A1, May 1917, pp. 44–5

64 McKernan, Michael, *The Australian People and the Great War*, Collins, Sydney, 1984, p. 128; Bishop, James, *Social History of the First World War*, Angus & Robertson, London, 1982, p. 115

65 Scantlebury Brown, Vera, Diary letters, vol. A12, July 1918, p. 1–14, vol. A10, March 1918, p. 37

66 Scantlebury Brown, Vera, Diary letters, vol. A7, October 1917, p. 35

67 Scantlebury Brown, Vera, Diary letters, vol. A4, July 1917, p. 63

68 Beckett, Ian, *Home Front 1914–1918: How Britain Survived the Great War*, National Archives, London, 2006, pp. 182–4

69 Scantlebury Brown, Vera, Diary letters, vol. A6, September 1917, p. 47

70 Woollacott, Angela, *To Try Her Fortune in London: Australian Women, Colonialism and Modernity*, Oxford University Press, 2001, pp. 32, 167

71 Woollacott, *To Try Her Fortune in London*, p. 167; McMullin, Ross, *Farewell Dear People: Biographies of Australia's Lost Generation*, Scribe, Melbourne, 2012, p. 393

72 'Bage, Jessie Eleanor', *Australian Women's Biographical Register*, www.womenaustralia.info/biogs; Scantlebury Brown, Vera, Diary letters, vol. A3, c. mid-May 1917, pp. 4, 22

73 Scantlebury Brown, Vera, Diary letters, vol. A8, January 1918, p. 79

Chapter 5: 'The brightest link in our love-chain broken'

1 Letter from Mary De Garis, Ostrovo, to Mrs Russell, Edinburgh, in McLaren, Eva Shaw, *A History of the Scottish Women's Hospitals*, General Books LLC, Memphis, 2012, p. 74

2 Dr Alice Benham, *Sydney Morning Herald*, 5 July 1917. Dr Benham was with Dr Forster and the BFH in the Belgium retreat in late 1914.

3 *British Journal of Nursing*, 27 October 1917, p. 269

4   Cherkasov, A, Metreveli, R, Smigel, M & Malchanova, V, 'Characteristics of the Russian Society of the Red Cross on the Caucasus Front (1914–1917)', *Terra Sebus, Acta Musei Sabesiensis*, vol. 8, 2016, p. 319

5   'The Indefatigable Florence MacDowell', www.awm.gov.au/blog/2009/03/05/the-indefatigable-florence-macdowell/

6   *British Journal of Nursing*, 20 January 1917, p. 51

7   Ibid., p. 102

8   Ibid., p. 104

9   De Garis, *Clinical Notes and Deductions*, p. 158

10   Ibid.

11   Letters from Mary De Garis, Ostrovo, to Mrs Russell, Edinburgh, various correspondence, 1917–18, SWH Archive, Mitchell Library, Glasgow

12   Agnes Bennett in McLaren, *A History of the Scottish Women's Hospitals*, p. 263

13   McLaren, *A History of the Scottish Women's Hospitals*, p. 400

14   De Garis, *Clinical Notes and Deductions*, p. 100

15   Ibid., p. 113

16   Williams, *No Easy Path*, p. 71

17   Ibid., p. 71

18   Manson & Manson, *Doctor Agnes Bennett*, p. 113

19   Franklin, Miles, '*Ne Mari Nishta:* Six Months with the Serbs', unpublished manuscript, ML MSS6035/7, Mitchell Library, State Library of New South Wales, p. 82

20   Letter from Mary De Garis, Ostrovo, to Bessie De Garis, Broadford, 11 June 1917, Mary De Garis Papers

21   McLaren, *A History of the Scottish Women's Hospitals*, p. 75

22   De Garis, *Clinical Notes and Deductions*, p. 154

23   'WWI Australian soldiers and nurses who rest in the United Kingdom: Alec Gustavus Sim', http://ww1austburialsuk.weebly.com/uploads/4/9/7/8/4978039/sim_alec_gustavus.pdf

24   The Medical Front, 'Extract from The Medical Department of the United States in the World War, Vol XIV, Medical Aspects of Gas Warfare', www.vlib.us/medical/gaswar/gas.htm

25   *The Argus*, 7 June, 1919, p. 11

26   'Royal Herbert Pavilions', www.royalherbert.co.uk/history.php

27   Bagnold, Enid, *A Diary Without Dates*, William Heinemann, London, 1918, p. 71. Enid Bagnold worked as a VAD at the Royal

Herbert Hospital in 1917. A *char-à-banc* was an elongated horse-drawn or motorised vehicle generally used for outings and could hold 12–14 people.

28   1st AIF Personnel Records 1914–1920, Series B2455, 'Ronald Lennox Henderson', www.naa.gov.au/collection/explore/defence/service-records

29   Bagnold, *A Diary Without Dates*, p. 45

30   Scantlebury Brown, Vera, Papers, vol. A2, 24 May 1917, p. 90; vol. A9, 14 February 1918, p. 30

31   Scantlebury Brown, Vera, Papers and memorabilia, 2013.0058, 1906–1936

32   *AIF Unit War Diaries 1914–1918 War*, Australian Light Horse Regiment Item No. 10/15/21, 10 March 1917, Australian War Memorial, Canberra

33   *The Observer*, 3 February, 1917, p. 28

34   Scantlebury Brown, Vera, Diary letters, vol. A1, 6 March 1917, p. 1

35   Ibid., p. 3

36   Ibid., p. 17

37   Kovac, Anthony, 'Choice of Anesthetic Technique for Surgery at the Front during World War I', *Journal of Anesthetisia History*, vol. 26, issue 1, 2008, www.anesthesiahistoryjournal.org/article/S1522-8649(08)50002-3/pdf

38   Vera's letters home took the form of books with carbon sheets. The top copy was posted to Australia and the books retained. Between March 1917 and February 1919 she filled 19 volumes. They are held in the archives of the Baillieu Library, University of Melbourne.

39   Scantlebury Brown, Vera, Diary letters, vol. A3, June 1917, p. 25

40   Butler, AG, *Official History of the Australian Army Medical Corps*, Australian War Memorial, Melbourne, 1943, p. 306

41   Scantlebury Brown, Vera, Diary letters, vol. A2, May 1917, p. 33

42   Sheard, Heather, 'A Heart Undivided, A Biographical Study of Dr Vera Scantlebury Brown, 1889–1946', PhD Thesis, School of Philosophical & Historical Studies, University of Melbourne, 2012, p. 64

43   Scantlebury Brown, Vera, Diary letters, vol. A3, June 1917, p. 68

44   Scantlebury Brown, Vera, Diary letters, vol. A7, 24 October 1917, pp. 48, 50

45   Scantlebury Brown, Vera, Diary letters, vol. A8, January 1918, p. 70

46 At the hospital, doctors were always addressed military-style, by their family name. Vera Scantlebury's letters refer to 'Bourne' and to 'Hamilton-Browne' but she makes an exception for her close friend Rachel Champion, always referring to her as 'Ray'.

47 Scantlebury Brown, Vera, Diary letters, vol. A2, 6 May 1917, p. 39

48 Scantlebury Brown, Vera, Diary letters, 84/82, vol. A8, 14 January 1918, p. 70

49 Scantlebury Brown, Vera, Diary letters, vol. A9, 28 February 1918, p. 55

50 Scantlebury Brown, Vera, Diary letters, vol. A2, 30 April 1917, p. 25

51 1st AIF Personnel Records 1914–1920, Series B2455, 'Norman John Bullen', www.naa.gov.au/collection/explore/defence/service-records/

52 Cooter, Robert, Presentation to the South Australian Medical Heritage Society, 9 September 2009, www.samhs.org.au/Virtual%20Museum/Notable-individuals/chapple/chapple.html

53 For example, *Daily Herald*, 2 February 1916, p. 4; *The Journal*, 21 October 1916, p. 5

54 *The Register*, 3 September 1919, p. 7

55 Cowper, JM, *A Short History of Queen Mary's Army Auxiliary Corps*, Women's Royal Army Corps Association, London, 1967, p. 17

56 BBC Schools, World War One, *Life on the Frontline*, www.bbc.co.uk/schools/0/ww1/25826265

57 Bowen, Claire, 'WAACs: Crossing the Line in the Great War', *Miranda*, February 2010, pp. 4, 8

58 *The Register*, 3 September 1919, p. 7

59 'Dr. Dalyell', *The Magazine of the Women's College*, vol. 7, 1920, p. 11

60 Little, Marjory, 'Some Pioneer Medical Women of the University of Sydney', Annual Post-Graduate Oration, University of Sydney, 1958, p. 47

61 Scantlebury Brown, Vera, Diary letters, vol. A6, September 1917, p. 57

Chapter 6: 'The very uselessness and waste of it all'

1 Scantlebury Brown, Vera, Diary letters, vol. AN3, April 1918, p. 90

2 Barry, JM, 'The Site of the Origin of the 1918 Influenza Pandemic and Its Public Health Implications', *Journal of Translational Medicine*, vol. 2, January 2004

3 Shanks, GD & Brundage, JF, 'Pathogenic Responses among Young Adults during the 1918 Influenza Pandemic', *Journal of Emerging Infectious Diseases*, vol. 18, 2, February 2012, p. 202

4   Manson & Manson, *Dr Agnes Bennett*, p. 114

5   Elston, MA, 'Fairfield, (Josephine) Letitia Denny, 1885–1978', *Oxford Dictionary of National Biography*, Oxford University Press, 2004

6   *Sydney Morning Herald*, 11 November 1914, p. 5

7   Eleanor Elizabeth Bourne Papers, State Library of Queensland, SLQ OM81-130, p. 7

8   *The Weekly Times*, 23 March 1918, p. 9

9   *The Register*, 3 September 1919, p. 7

10   Bowen, Claire, 'WAAC's: Crossing the Line in the Great War', *Miranda*, vol. 2, 2010, pp. 5–6, 8

11   Cowper, JM, *A Short History of Queen Mary's Army Auxiliary Corps*, Women's Royal Army Corps Association, pp. 52–3

12   'Alice Thomasson', http://Gm1914.wordpress.com/2016/11/10/alice-thomasson/

13   Special Supplement to the *London Gazette*, 18 October 1918, No. 30962

14   *The Register*, 3 September 1919, p. 7

15   'Historical College Roll: Little, Elaine Marjory', www.racp.edu.au/about/library/historical-college-roll/

16   'Marjory Little', *Medical Journal of Australia*, vol. 2, 1974, pp. 338–9

17   The first director designate was Dr Gordon Clunes Mathieson but he was wounded at Cape Helles, Gallipoli, on 9 May 1915 and died in hospital in Alexandria on 18 May 1915.

18   Patterson, SW, 'The Pathology of Influenza in France', *Medical Journal of Australia*, vol. 1, 6 March 1920, p. 5

19   Little, Elaine Marjory, 'Obituary: Fanny [sic] Eleanor Williams', *Medical Journal of Australia*, 9 November 1963, p. 811

20   'Aubrey Cumberbatch, British West Indies Regiment', Cumberbatch family history, http://cumberbatch.one-name.net/getperson.php?personID=I9679&tree=001

21   Snowden, Betty, 'Iso Rae in Étaples, Another Perspective of War', *Wartime*, vol. 8, Summer 1999, p. 37

22   Gillings, J & Richards, J (eds), *In All These Lines: The Diary of Sister Elsie Tranter, 1916–1919*, Gillings & Richards, Newstead Tasmania, 2011, http://throughtheselines.com.au/research/étaples

23   Ibid.

24   Marjory Little, 'Life in a Lab in France', *Sydney University Medical Journal*, vol. XVII, Part 1, May 1923, p. 20

25   Snowden, 'Iso Rae in Étaples', p. 38

26 Little, 'Life in a Lab in France', p. 18
27 Ibid.
28 Letter from Colonel SL Cummins to Lieutenant Colonel C Martin, 1919, in 'Marjory Little', *Medical Journal of Australia*, vol. 2, 1974, pp. 338–9
29 Private correspondence from Pacita Alexander, 7 June 2014
30 Bishop, Alan & Bostridge, Mark (eds), *Letters from a Lost Generation, First World War Letters of Vera Brittain and Four Friends*, Abacus, London, 1999, p. 371
31 *Sydney Morning Herald*, 29 May 1918, p. 11

Chapter 7: 'This wholesale slaughter cannot go on forever'

1   Scantlebury Brown, Vera, Diary letters, vol. A10, May 1918, p. 85
2   Ibid., p. 22
3   Photograph of No. 19 British General Hospital, Australian War Memorial, www.awm.gov.au/collection/A02858
4   Smythe, Percy, 'The World War I Diary of Percy Smythe', www.smythe.id.au/diary/ch1.htm
5   Butler, AG, *Official History of Australian Army Medical Services*, Australian War Memorial, 1943, p. 765
6   Leneman, Leah, 'Medical Women at War, 1914–1918', *Medical History*, vol. 38, 1994, p. 171
7   Butler, *Official History of Australian Army Medical Services*, pp. 752, 764
8   Sergeant Major, RAMC, *With the RAMC in Egypt*, Cassell & Company, London 1918, p. 81
9   Mortlock, Michael, *The Egyptian Expeditionary Force in World War One: A History of the British-led Campaigns in Egypt, Palestine & Syria*, MacFarland & Co, Jefferson, North Carolina, p. 63
10 Shanks, G Dennis, 'Simultaneous Epidemics of Influenza and Malaria in the Australian Army in Palestine in 1918', *Medical Journal of Australia*, vol. 191, no.11, 2009, p. 656
11 Letter from EC De Garis, Guernsey, to Mary De Garis, Ostrovo, 12 June 1918, Mary De Garis Papers, privately held
12 Letter from Ostrovo staff to Mrs Laurie, Administrator, SWH, Edinburgh, June 1918 in Lee, *Woman War Doctor*, p. 100
13 De Garis, *Clinical Notes*, p. 170–71
14 Bennett, 'With the Serbians', *Sydney Morning Herald*, p. 6.
15 Mary De Garis, London, to Mrs Laurie, Edinburgh, 9 December 1918, Personnel files, Tin 36, Mitchell Library, Glasgow

16   For a full description of the award, see Lee, *Woman War Doctor*,
     p. 169
17   Lee, *Woman War Doctor*, pp. 105,106.
18   Scantlebury Brown, Vera, Diary letters, vol. A11, May 1918, p. 33
19   Elston, MA, 'Fairfield, (Josephine) Letitia Denny (1885–1978)',
     Oxford Dictionary of National Biography, Oxford University Press,
     2004
20   'Obituary L Fairfield', *British Medical Journal*, 11 February 1978,
     p. 873
21   Garrett, Emily, *A Woman of Some Importance*, http://blog.
     wellcomelibrary.org/2014/10/a-woman-of-some-importance
22   Atkinson, Diane, *Elsie & Mairi Go to War: Two Extraordinary Women
     on the Western Front*, Arrow Books, London, 2009, p. 198
23   Fairfield, Letitia, 'Medical Women in the Forces 1914–1918 War',
     Journal of the Medical Women's Federation, vol. 49, 1967, p. 99
24   'Buildings at Risk Register for Scotland: Bangour Village Hospital',
     www.buildingsatrisk.org.uk/details/960257
25   Elsie Tranter quoted in De Vries, Susanna, *Australian Heroines of
     World War One, Gallipoli, Lemnos and the Western Front*, Pirgos Press,
     Brisbane, 2013, p. 370
26   Scantlebury Brown, Vera, Diary letters, vol. A14, October 1918,
     pp. 8, 10
27   Ibid., p. 18
28   *Western Argus*, 3 February 1920, p. 27
29   *The Argus*, 27 February 1920, p. 7
30   Little, E Marjory, 'Dysentery: Bacillary & Amoebic', *Medical Journal
     of Australia*, vol. 1, 6 June 1923, p. 1

Chapter 8: 'By gosh! It's peace!'

1   Scantlebury Brown, Vera, Diary letters, vol. A14, October 1918,
     p. 50
2   Manson & Manson, *Dr Agnes Bennett*, p. 118
3   Scantlebury Brown, Vera, Diary letters, vol. A14, October 1918, p. 50
4   Ibid., p. 57
5   *The Common Cause*, 3 December 1915, p. 450
6   Murray, Flora, 'The Position of Women in Medicine and Surgery',
     New Statesman, vol. 1, 20 April 1913, pp. xvi–xvii
7   Scantlebury Brown, Vera, Diary letters, vol. A10, May 1918, p. 92;
     Mellor, *150 Years, 150 Firsts*, p. 14

8   O'Riordan, JLH, 'Rickets, from History to Molecular Biology, from Monkeys to YACS', *Journal of Endocrinology*, no. 154, 1997, p. 53

9   Alexander, Wendy, *First Ladies of Medicine*, Wellcome Unit for the History of Medicine, Glasgow, 1987, p. 56; Leneman, 'Medical Women at War', p. 176

10   Hutton, Isabel Emslie, *Memories of a Doctor in War and Peace*, Heinemann, London, 1960, p. 177

11   *Sydney Morning Herald*, 26 September 1914, p. 3

12   Private correspondence from Pacita Alexander, 7 June 2014

13   Little, Marjory, 'Some Pioneer Medical Women of the University of Sydney', Annual Post-Graduate Oration, University of Sydney, 1958, p. 7

Biographical notes

1   Radi, Heather, 'Ardill, Katie Louisa (1886–1955)', *Australian Dictionary of Biography*, National Centre of Biography, Australian National University, http://adb.anu.edu.au/biography/ardill-katie-louisa-5624/text8413

2   Private correspondence from Dr Baker's extended family

3   Private correspondence from Dr Baker's extended family

4   1st AIF Personnel Records, 1914–1920, Series B2455, 'Richard Hamilton Baker', www.naa.gov.au/collection/explore/defence/service-records

5   Wagner, RL, 'Dr Laura Elizabeth Forster', *Sabretache*, vol. LVIII, no. 4, December 1917, p. 33

6   Fairfield, L, 'Medical Women in the Forces, Part 1, Women Doctors in the British Forces, 1914–1918 War,' *Journal of the Medical Women's Federation*, no. 49, 1967, p. 99.

7   'A Successful Lady Student', *The Hebrew Standard of Australasia*, Sydney, 12 July 1905, p. 5

8   'Personal', *The Mercury* (Hobart), 13 May 1918, p. 4

9   'Obituary Dr Eveline Cohen', *The Hebrew Standard of Australasia*, Sydney, 24 March 1922, p. 7

10   Brookes, Barbara, 'A Corresponding Community: Dr Agnes Bennett and her Friends from the Edinburgh Medical College for Women of the 1890s,' *Medical History*, vol. 52, 2008, p. 237

11   Manson & Manson, *Dr Agnes Bennett*, p. 113

12   Ibid, p. 119

13 Bell, Jacqueline, 'Bourne, Eleanor Elizabeth (1878–1957)', *Australian Dictionary of Biography*, vol. 7, Melbourne University Press, 1979, p. 356

14 Williams, *No Better Profession*, pp.13–14

15 Bell, 'Bourne, Eleanor Elizabeth (1878–1957)', p. 356.

16 Ibid.

17 Eleanor Elizabeth Bourne Papers, State Library of Queensland, SLQ OM81-130, p. 1

18 Likeman, Robert, *Australian Doctors on the Western Front: France and Belgium 1916–1918*, Rosenberg Publications, Sydney, 2014, p. 473

19 Ibid.

20 Gibbney, HJ & Smith, Ann G (eds), *A Biographical Register 1788–1939*, Volume 1: Notes from the name index of the Australian Dictionary of Biography, ANU, 1987, p. 94; Neve, M Hutton, *This Mad Folly: The History of Australia's Pioneer Women Doctors*, Library of Australian History, Sydney, 1980, p. 241

21 *Sydney Morning Herald*, 19 January 1933, p. 3

22 Walker, DR, 'Esson, Thomas Louis Buvelot (1878–1943)', *Australian Dictionary of Biography*, http://adb.anu.edu.au/biography/esson-thomas-louis-buvelot-6115

23 Fitzpatrick, Peter, *Pioneer Players: The Lives of Louis and Hilda Esson*, Cambridge University Press, Melbourne, 1995, p. 147–8

24 Walker, 'Esson, Thomas Louis Buvelot (1878-1943)'

25 *Argus* (Melbourne), 30 June 1953, p. 5

26 Likeman, *Australian Doctors on the Western Front*, p. 1945

27 Unpublished family history, 'Which Way's Home', Shaw family archive, privately held

28 Scantlebury Brown, Vera, Diary letters, vol. A2, May 1917, p. 52

29 Blanch, Craig, 'Dr Phoebe Chapple: The First Woman Doctor to Win the Military Medal', Australian War Memorial, 2009, www.awm.gov.au/articles/blog/dr-phoebe-chapple-the-first-woman-doctor-to-receive-the-military-medal

30 Gibberd, Joyce, 'Chapple, Phoebe (1879–1967)', *Australian Dictionary of Biography*, http://adb.anu.edu.au/biography/chapple-phoebe-5560

31 'From War to Peace: Dr Phoebe Chapple's Return', *The Register* (Adelaide), 3 September 1919, p.7

32 Ibid.

33   Williams, *No Easy Path*, p. 76
34   Cramond, T, 'Lilian Violet Cooper, MD, FRACS, Foundation Fellow, Royal Australasian College of Surgeons', *Australian and New Zealand Journal of Surgery*, vol. 63, 1993, p. 134
35   Leggett, CAC, 'Cooper, Lilian Violet (1861–1947)' *Australian Dictionary of Biography*, http://adb.anu.edu.au/biography/cooper-lilian-violet-5770
36   Cramond, 'Lilian Violet Cooper, MD, FRACS', p. 135
37   Ibid., p. 136
38   Leggett, 'Cooper, Lilian Violet (1861–1947)'
39   Ibid.
40   Williams, *No Easy Path* , p. 76
41   Anonymous. *Queensland 1900 – A Narrative of Her Past, Together with Biographies of Her Leading Men*, Alcazar Press, Brisbane, 1900, p. 175, quoted in Cramond, p. 138
42   Cramond, 'Lilian Violet Cooper, MD, FRACS', pp. 137–8
43   Ibid., p. 136
44   Ibid., p. 138
45   Ibid., p. 139
46   Likeman, *Australian Doctors on the Western Front*, p. 1962
47   *Australasian* (Melbourne), 14 September 1929, p. 14
48   *Medical Journal of Australia*, 13 September 1958, vol. II, no. 11, p. 348
49   Service Record of Elsie Jean Dalyell, *Lady Doctors of the Malta Garrison*, www.maltaramc.com/ladydoc/d/dalyellej.html
50   Ibid.
51   Mitchell, Ann M, 'Dalyell, Elsie Jean (1881–1948)', *Australian Dictionary of Biography*, http://adb.anu.edu.au/biography/dalyell-elsie-jean-5875
52   Ibid.
53   Richardson, GD, *The Dalyells and Their Kin: A Chronicle of a family*, 2nd edition, GD Richardson, Canberra, 2010
54   Neve, *This Mad Folly*, p. 7
55   Mitchell, Ann M, 'Dalyell, Elsie Jean (1881–1948)', *Australian Dictionary of Biography*, Vol. 8, MUP 1981, http://adb.anu.edu.au/biography/dalyell-elsie-jean-5875
56   Mary De Garis Papers, privately held
57   Lee, *Woman War Doctor*, p. 154
58   'Obituary', *British Medical Journal*, 21 August 1920, p. 298

59   'Victorians in Europe', *The Prahran Telegraph*, 21 February 1914, p. 1
60   'Dr Irene C. Davey Eaton', *British Medical Journal*, 21 August 1920, p. 293
61   Elston, MA, 'Fairfield, (Josephine) Letitia Denny (1885–1978)'
62   Ibid.
63   Ibid.
64   Ryde City Council, 'Brush Farm House', www.ryde.nsw.gov.au/Library/Local-and-Family-History/Historic-Ryde/Historic-Buildings/Brush-Farm-House
65   *The Daily News* (Western Australia), 16 October, 1918, p. 4
66   Cleese, Mary & Cleese, Thomas, *Ladies in the Laboratory III: South African, Australian, New Zealand and Canadian Women in Science: 19th and Early 20th Centuries, A Survey of Their Contributions*, The Scare Crow Press, Plymouth, 2010, p. 64
67   *Sydney Morning Herald*, 16 May 1917, p. 7
68   Ibid.
69   Cleese & Cleese, *Ladies in the Laboratory III*, p. 75
70   *Sydney Morning Herald*, 5 July 1917, p. 6
71   Ibid.
72   Likeman, *Australian Doctors on the Western Front*, p. 1967
73   Jones, Helen 'Hope, Laura Margaret (1868–1952)', http://adb.anu.edu.au/biography/hope-laura-margaret-10541
74   Ibid.
75   Alafaci, Annette, 'Gullett, Edith Lucy (1876–1949)', *The Australian Women's Register*, www.womenaustralia.info/biogs/AWE1829b.htm
76   Ibid.
77   Swain, Shurlee 'Gullett, Lucy Edith', *The Encyclopedia of Women and Leadership in Twentieth Century Australia*, www.womenaustralia.info/leaders/biogs/WLE0123b.htm
78   Neve, *This Mad Folly*, p. 7
79   Ibid.
80   *Sydney Morning Herald*, 18 November 1949, p. 2
81   *Sydney Morning Herald* 18 September 1931, p. 10
82   *Sydney Morning Herald*, 18 November 1949, p. 2
83   Cohen, Susan L, 'Hamilton, Lillias Anna (1858–1925)', *Oxford Dictionary of National Biography*, Oxford University Press, 2004
84   'Dr Lillias Hamilton: Adventure and Service', Obituary, *The Times*, London, 9 January 1925
85   Hoyle, *Flowers in the Snow*, p. 25

86 Ibid., p. 82

87 'Dr Lillias Hamilton: Adventure and Service', *The Times*

88 Prosectors prepare dissections on a human corpse for the purposes of demonstration in medical anatomy schools.

89 'Elizabeth Hamilton-Browne', Early Women Students, ARMS, University of Sydney, http://sydney.edu.au/arms/archives/history/students_early_women_HamiltonBrowne.shtml

90 *Daily Mirror*, 31 July 1985, p. 13.

91 Likeman, *Australian Doctors on the Western Front*, p. 157

92 Heagney, Brenda, 'Little, Elaine Marjory (1884–1974*)*', *Australian Dictionary of Biography*, http://adb.anu.edu.au/biography/little-elaine-marjory-10838

93 'Obituary: Elaine Marjory Little', *Pathology Journal*, vol. 7, no. 3, 1975, p. 259

94 Heagney, 'Little, Elaine Marjory (1884–1974)', *Australian Dictionary of Biography*

95 'Marjory Little', *Medical Journal of Australia*, vol. 2, 1974, p. 339

96 *The Telegraph* (Brisbane), 21 January 1932, p. 15

97 Cousins, Arthur and Hall, George, *Book of Remembrance of the University of Sydney in the Great War, 1914–1918*, 'Mabel Murray-Prior', 1939, University of Sydney, as cited on: http://beyond1914.sydney.edu.au/profile/3705/mabel-murray-prior

98 Ibid.

99 *Telegraph* (Brisbane), 21 January 1932, p. 15

100 Annable, Rosemary, *The Women's College Biographical Register, vol. 1, 1892–1939*, Council of the Women's College, Sydney, 1995–2007, p. 40

101 *Leader* (Orange), 30 April 1920, p. 3; *Daily Post Hobart*, 12 August 1910, p. 4

102 McQuellin, Christopher, 'Dr Isabel Ormiston', *Albury & District Historical Society Bulletin*, no. 541, December 2013, p. 5

103 *Table Talk*, 12 March 1919, p. 9

104 McQuellin, 'Doctor Isabel Ormiston', p. 5

105 Sheard, *A Heart Undivided*, pp. 3–4

106 Geddes, 'Women as Army Surgeons', pp. 2, 33–5

107 Sheard, *A Heart Undivided*, pp. 116–18

108 Waters, Joan, *Changing Minds, Changing Lives: The Legacy of the Vera Scantlebury Brown Memorial Trust 1946-2004*, Department of Paediatrics, University of Melbourne, Parkville, 2010

109 Russell, Penny, 'Sexton, Hannah Mary Helen (1862–1950)', *Australian Dictionary of Biography* online edition, http://adb.anu.edu.au/biography/sexton-hannah-mary-helen-8389

110 McCalman, Janet, *Sex and Suffering: Women's Health and a Women's Hospital*, Melbourne University Press, 1998, p. 86

111 Russell, 'Sexton, Hannah Mary Helen (1862–1950)'

112 Ibid.

113 *The Age*, 1 December 1934, p. 19

114 Reiger, Kerreen, 'Ross, Isabella Henrietta Younger (Isie) (1887–1956)', *Australian Dictionary of Biography*, adb.anu.edu.au/biography/ross-isabella-henrietta-younger-isie-8272

115 Pritchard, Eric, *The Infant, Nutrition & Management*, Edward Arnold, London, 1913

116 Younger Ross, Isabella, *Baby Health*, vol. 1, no. 11, December 1950

117 Sheard, *All the Little Children, The Story of Victoria's Baby Health Centres*, 2nd edition, Maternal Child Health Nurses Victoria, Melbourne, 2017, p. 18–19, 26–28

Bibliography

Books

Alexander, Wendy, *First Ladies of Medicine*, Wellcome Unit for the History of Medicine, Glasgow, 1987

Annable, Rosemary, *The Women's College Biographical Register*, vol. 1, 1892–1939, Council of the Women's College, Sydney, 1995–2007

Atkinson, Diane, *Elsie & Mairi Go To War: Two Extraordinary Women on the Western Front*, Arrow Books, London, 2009

Australian Dictionary of Biography, Melbourne University Press, 1981

Bagnold, Enid, *A Diary Without Dates*, William Heinemann, London, 1918

Barrett, JW & Dean, PE, *The AAMC in Egypt*, HK Lewis, London, 1918

Barwick, Archie, *In Great Spirits: Archie Barwick's WWI Diary*, HarperCollins, Sydney, 2013

Bassett, Jan, *Guns and Brooches: Australian Army Nursing from the Boer War to the Gulf War*, Oxford University Press, Melbourne, 1992

Beaumont, Joan, *Broken Nation: Australians in the Great War*, Allen & Unwin, Sydney, 2013

Beckett, Ian, *Home Front 1914–1918: How Britain Survived the Great War*, National Archives, London, 2006

Bishop, Alan & Bostridge, Mark (eds), *Letters from a Lost Generation: First World War Letters of Vera Brittain and Four Friends*, Abacus, London, 1999

Bishop, James, *Social History of the First World War*, Angus & Robertson, London, 1982

Bowerbank, Major, *New Zealand Hospitals in Egypt: The War Effort of New Zealand*, Whitcomb & Tombs, Auckland, 1923

Brittain, Vera, *Testament of Youth*, Wideview Books, USA, 1980

Butler, AG, *Official History of the Australian Army Medical Corps*, Australian War Memorial, Melbourne, 1943

Clark, Matilda Emily, *A War Nurse's Diary: Sketches from a Belgian Field Hospital*, The Macmillan Company, New York, 1918

Clayton, Anthony, *Paths of Glory: The French Army 1914–1918*, Cassell, London, 2003

Cleese, Mary & Cleese, Thomas, *Ladies in the Laboratory III: South African, Australian, New Zealand and Canadian Women in Science: 19th and Early 20th Centuries, A Survey of their Contributions*, The Scare Crow Press, Plymouth, 2010

Cohen, Susan, *Medical Services in the First World War*, Shire Publications, Oxford, 2014

Cowper, Julia Margaret, *A Short History of Queen Mary's Army Auxiliary Corps*, Women's Royal Army Corps Association, London, 1967

Creswick, P, Pond, G & Ashton, P, *Kent's Care for the Wounded*, Hodder & Stoughton, London, 1915

Crofton, Eileen, *The Women of Royaumont: A Scottish Women's Hospital on the Western Front*, Tuckwell Press, East Lothian, 1997

De Garis, MC, *Clinical Notes and Deductions of a Peripatetic: Being Fads and Fancies of a General Practitioner*, Bailliere, Tindall and Cox, London, 1926

De Vries, Susanna, *Australian Heroines of World War One, Gallipoli, Lemnos and the Western Front*, Pirgos Press, Brisbane, 2013

Edwards, Nina, *Dressed for War: Uniform, Civilian Clothing & Trappings, 1914–1918*, LB Tauris & Co, London, 2014

Englund, Peter, *The Beauty and the Sorrow: An Intimate History of the First World War*, Profile Books, London, 2010

Fitzpatrick, Peter, *Pioneer Players: The Lives of Louis and Hilda Esson*, Cambridge University Press, Melbourne, 1995

Gammage, Bill, *The Broken Years: Australian Soldiers in the Great War*, Australian National University Press, Canberra, 1974

Gatrell, Peter & Zuanko, Livbov (eds), *Europe on the Move: Refugees in the Era of the Great War*, Manchester Universty Press, 2017

Gillings, J & Richards, J (eds), *In All these Lines: The Diary of Sister Elsie Tranter, 1916–1919*, Gillings & Richards, Newstead Tasmania, 2011

Grayzel, Susan, *Women and the First World War*, Longman, London, 2002

Hallam, Andrew & Hallam, Nicola (eds), *Lady Under Fire on the Western Front: The Great War Letters of Lady Dorothie Feilding MM*, Pen & Sword Books, Yorkshire, 2011

Hallett, Christine, *Veiled Warriors: Allied Nurses of the First World War*, Oxford University Press, Oxford, 2014

Harris, Kirsty, *More Than Bombs and Bandages: Australian Army Nurses at Work in World War I*, Big Sky Publishing, Newport, 2011

Hoyle, Gwyneth, *Flowers in the Snow*, University of Nebraska Press, Lincoln, 2001

Hutton, Isabel Emslie, *Memories of a Doctor in War and Peace*, Heinemann, London, 1960

Johnston, Olive (ed), *The Hands of a Woman*, Wakefield Press, Adelaide, 1994

Kent, Susan Kingsley, *Making Peace: The Reconstruction of Gender in Interwar Britain*, Princeton University, Princeton, 1993

King-Hall, Stephen, *A North Sea Diary 1914–1918*, Newnes, London, 1936

Krippner, Monica, *The Quality of Mercy, Women at War, 1915–1918*, David & Charles, London, 1980

Lee, Ruth L, *Woman War Doctor: The Life of Mary De Garis*, Australian Scholarly Publishing, Melbourne, 2014

Leneman, Leah, *In the Service of Life: The Story of Elsie Inglis and the Scottish Women's Hospitals*, Mercat Press, Edinburgh, 1994

Likeman, Robert, *Australian Doctors on the Western Front: France and Belgium 1916–1918*, Rosenberg Publications, Sydney, 2014

Maclean, Hester, *Nursing in New Zealand: History and Reminiscences*, Tolan Printing Company, 1932

Manson, Cecil & Manson, Celia, *Dr Agnes Bennett*, Michael Joseph, London, 1960

Marlow, Joyce (ed), *The Virago Book of Women in the Great War*, Virago, London, 2011

Mayhew, Emily, *Wounded: A New History of the Western Front in World War I*, Oxford University Press, New York, 2014

McCalman, Janet, *Sex and Suffering: Women's Health and a Women's Hospital*, Melbourne University Press, 1998

McKernan, Michael, *The Australian People and the Great War*, Collins, Sydney, 1984

McLaren, Eva Shaw, *A History of the Scottish Women's Hospitals*, General Books LLC, Memphis, 2012

McMullin, Ross, *Farewell Dear People: Biographies of Australia's Lost Generation*, Scribe, Melbourne, 2012

Mellor, Lise, *150 Years, 150 Firsts: The People of the Faculty of Medicine*, Sydney University Press, 2006

Miles, Hallie, *Untold Tales of War-Time London: A Personal Diary*, Cecil Palmer, London, 1930

Mitchell, Ann M, 'Medical Women and the Medical Services

of the First World War' in *Festschrift for Kenneth Fitzpatrick Russell: Proceedings of a Symposium arranged by the Section of Medical History, AMA (Victorian Branch)*, Queensberry Hill Press, Melbourne, 1978

Mitchell, David, *Monstrous Regiment: The Story of the Women of the First World War*, The Macmillan Company, New York, 1965

Mortlock, Michael, *The Egyptian Expeditionary Force in World War One: A History of the British-led Campaigns in Egypt, Palestine & Syria*, MacFarland & Co, Jefferson, North Carolina, 2010

Murray, Flora, *Women as Army Surgeons*, 1st edition, Hodder & Stoughton, London, c. 1920

Murray, Flora, *Women as Army Surgeons*, 2nd edition, Cambridge University Press, London, 2014

Official Year Book of the Commonwealth of Australia, Commonwealth Government, 1918

Oxford Dictionary of National Biography, Oxford University Press, 2004

Neve, M Hutton, *This Mad Folly: The History of Australia's Pioneer Women Doctors*, Library of Australian History, Sydney, 1980

Plowman, Peter, *Across the Sea to War: Australian and New Zealand Troopships from 1865*, Rosenberg Publishing, Sydney, 2003

Powell, Anne, *Women in the War Zone: Hospital Service in the First World War*, The History Press, Gloucestershire, 2009

Pritchard, Eric, *The Infant: Nutrition & Management*, Edward Arnold, London, 1913

Proctor, Tammy, *Civilians in a World at War*, New York University Press, New York, 2010

Reznick, Jeffrey, *Healing the Nation: Soldiers and the Culture of Care Giving in Britain During the Great War*, Manchester University Press, 2004

Richardson, GD, *The Dalyells and Their Kin: A Chronicle of a Family*, 2nd edition, GD Richardson, Canberra, 2010

Sergeant Major, RAMC, *With the RAMC in Egypt*, Cassell & Company, London 1918

Sheard, Heather, *A Heart Undivided: The Life of Dr Vera Scantlebury Brown, 1889–1946*, Faculty of Medicine, Dentistry and Health Sciences, University of Melbourne, 2016

Sheard, Heather, *All the Little Children, The Story of Victoria's Baby Health Centres*, 2nd edition, Maternal Child Health Nurses Victoria, Melbourne, 2017

Sinclair, May, *A Journal of Impressions in Belgium*, The Macmillan Company, New York, 1915

Smith, Angela, *British Women of the Eastern Front*, Manchester University Press, Manchester, 2016

Souttar, Henry Sessions, *A Surgeon in Belgium*, Edward Arnold, London, 1915

Stebbing, EP, *At the Serbian Front in Macedonia*, John Lane, London, 1917

Storr, Katherine, *Excluded from the Record: Women, Refugees and Relief, 1914–1929*, Peter Lang, Bern, 2010

Tilton, May, *The Grey Battalion*, Angus & Robertson, Sydney, 1933

Tudor, Spencer (ed), *World War I: Encyclopedia Vol 1*, ABC-CLIO, Santa Barbara, 2005

Van Bergen, Leo, *Before My Helpless Sight: Suffering, Dying & Military Medicines on the Western Front 1914–1918*, Ashgate Publishing, Surrey, 1988

Walsh, Michael, *Brothers in War*, Random House, London, 2011

Waters, Joan, *Changing Minds, Changing Lives: The Legacy of the Vera Scantlebury Brown Memorial Trust 1946–2004*, Department of Paediatrics, University of Melbourne, Parkville, 2010

Williams, Lesley M, *No Better Profession: Medical Women in Queensland, 1891–1999*, Watson, Ferguson & Co, Brisbane, 2006

Williams, Lesley M, *No Easy Path: The Life and Times of Lilian Violet Cooper*, Department of Child Health Publishing Unit, Royal Children's Hospital, Brisbane, 1991

Winter, Jay & Robert, Jean-Louis, *Capital Cities at War: Paris, London, Berlin 1914–1919*, Cambridge University Press, New York, 2007

Woollacott, Angela, *To Try Her Fortune in London: Australian Women, Colonialism and Modernity*, Oxford University Press, New York, 2001

Woollacott, Angela, *Gender and Empire*, Palgrave Macmillan, London, 2006

Journal Articles

Barry, JM, 'The Site of the Origin of the 1918 Influenza Pandemic and Its Public Health Implications', *Journal of Translational Medicine*, vol. 2, January 2004

Bennett, Agnes, 'With Our Allies in the Balkans: Work of the Women's Hospital Units' (lecture), *Dominion*, vol. 11, issue 137, 27 February 1918

Bowen, Claire, 'WAACs: Crossing the Line in the Great War', *Miranda*, February 2010

Brookes, Barbara, 'A Corresponding Community: Dr Agnes Bennett and Her Friends from the Edinburgh Medical College for Women of the 1890s', *Medical History*, vol. 52, 2008

Cherkasov, A, Metreveli, R, Smigel, M & Malchanova, V, 'Characteristics of the Russian Society of the Red Cross on the Caucasus Front (1914–1917)', *Terra Sebus. Acta Musei Sabesiensis*, vol. 8, 2016

Cramond, Tess, 'Lilian Violet Cooper, MD, FRACS, Royal Australasian College of Surgeons', *Australia New Zealand Journal of Surgery*, No. 63, 1993

Dalyell, EJ, 'A Case of Gangrene Associated With B. Oedematics', *British Medical Journal*, 17 March 1917

Fairfield, L, 'Medical Women in the Forces, Part 1, Women Doctors in the British Forces, 1914–1918 War', *Journal of the Medical Women's Federation*, no. 49, 1967

Geddes, Jennian F, 'Deeds not Words in the Suffrage Military Hospital in Endell Street', *Medical History*, vol. 51, 1, 2007

Kovac, Anthony, 'Choice of Anesthetic Technique for Surgery at the Front during World War 1', *Journal of Anesthesia History*, vol. 26, issue 1, 2008

Lazovic, Ivana & Sujic, Radmila, 'Women Doctors in the Serbian Sanitary Service during the Balkan Wars', *Acta Medico-historica Adriatica*, vol. 5(1), 2007

Leneman, Leah, 'Medical Women at War, 1914–1918', *Medical History*, vol. 38, 1994

Little, E. Marjory 'Dysentery: Bacillary & Amoebic', *Medical Journal of Australia*, vol. 1, 6 June 1923

Little, Marjory, 'Life in a Lab in France', *Sydney University Medical Journal*, vol. XVII, Part 1, May 1923

Little, Marjory, 'Some Pioneer Medical Women of the University of Sydney', Annual Postgraduate Oration, University of Sydney, 1958

Maitland, Gwynne, 'Notes on the Typhus Epidemic in Serbia, 1915', *British Medical Journal*, 21 August 1915

O'Riordan, JLH, 'Rickets, from History to Molecular Biology, from Monkeys to YACS', *Journal of Endocrinology*, no. 154, 1997

Patterson, SW, 'The Pathology of Influenza in France', *Medical*

Journal of Australia, vol. 1, 6 March 1920

Secomb, Robin, 'Borne in Empire: Issues of Gender, Ethnicity and Power behind Laura Fowler Hope's Journey to Kalimpong', *Outskirts Online Journal*, vol. 7, November 2000

Shanks, GD, 'Simultaneous Epidemics of Influenza and Malaria in the Australian Army in Palestine in 1918', *Medical Journal of Australia*, vol. 191(11), 2009

Shanks, GD & Brundage, JF, 'Pathogenic Responses among Young Adults during the 1918 Influenza Pandemic', *Journal of Emerging Infectious Diseases*, vol. 18, no. 2, February 2012

Snowden, Betty, 'Iso Rae in Étaples, Another Perspective of War', *Wartime*, vol. 8, Summer 1999

Tschanz, David W, *Typhus Fever on the Eastern Front in World War I*, www.entomology.montana/edu/historybug/wwi

Wagner, RL, 'Dr Laura Elizabeth Forster', *Sabretache*, vol. LVIII, no. 4, December 2017

Weiner, MF, 'The Scottish Women's Hospital at Royaumont, France 1914–1919', *Journal of the Royal College of Physicians of Edinburgh*, vol. 44, 2014

'Women under Fire', *The British Journal of Nursing*, 17 October 1914

Wright, James R Jr & Baskin, Leland, 'Pathology and Laboratory Medicine Support for the American Expeditionary Forces by the US Army Medical Corps During World War I', *Archives of Pathology & Laboratory Medicine*, vol. 39, no. 9, Sept 2015

Newspapers and Periodicals

ADFA Health
Albury & District Historical Society Bulletin

Auckland Star
Baby Health – Victorian Baby Health Centres Association
Daily Herald
Daily Post (Hobart)
Evening Telegraph
Glen Innes Examiner
Hawera & Normanby Star
Jus Suffragii
Kai Teaki
Liverpool Daily Post
National Advocate
Nelson Evening Mail
New Statesman
Newcastle Journal
Queensland Figaro
Richmond River Herald
Singleton Argus
Sydney Morning Herald
Table Talk
The Age
The Argus
The British Australasian
The Common Cause
The Daily Mirror
The Great War
The Hebrew Standard of Australasia
The Leader (Orange)
The London Gazette
The Magazine of the Women's College of the University of Sydney
The Mercury
The Mirror Australia

The Register
The Times (London)
The Woman's World
Townsville Daily Bulletin
Warrnambool Standard
Wartime
Weekly Times
West Australian
Western Argus

Manuscripts and Personal Papers

'Account of America Unit', manuscript, Scottish Women's
    Hospitals, Imperial War Museum, London, BRCS 24.4/58
Agnes Elizabeth Lloyd Bennett, 1872–1960, MS-Papers-1346,
    Alexander Turnbull Library, National Library of New Zealand,
    Wellington, New Zealand
Eleanor Elizabeth Bourne Papers, State Library of Queensland,
    SLQ OM81-130
Mary De Garis Papers, privately held
Fowler Family Papers, PRG34, Mortlock Library of South
    Australia, State Library of South Australia, Adelaide
Miles Franklin, '*Ne Mari Nishta*: Six Months with the Serbs',
    unpublished manuscript, ML MSS6035/7, Mitchell Library,
    State Library of New South Wales
National Archives of Australia Personnel Service Records, World
    War I
Rachel Champion Shaw Papers, privately held
Vera Scantlebury Brown (1889–1946), University of Melbourne
    Archive, 1984.0082, 1917–1939; Papers & Memorabilia,

2013.0058, 1906–1936
Scottish Women's Hospital Archive, Mitchell Library, Glasgow, Scotland
Helen Sexton Casebook, Manuscript 2189, Australian Medical Association Archive, University of Melbourne Medical History Museum

Theses

Geddes, Jennian, 'Women as Army Surgeons: The Women's Hospital Corps', MA Thesis, London Metropolitan University, May 2005
Lee, Ruth L, 'Mary De Garis: Progressivism, Early Feminism and Medical Reform', PhD Thesis, Deakin University, 2010
McCarthy, Louella, 'Uncommon Practices: Medical Women in NSW 1885–1939', PhD Thesis, University of New South Wales, 2001
Sheard, Heather, 'A Heart Undivided: A Biographical Study of Dr Vera Scantlebury Brown, 1889–1946', PhD Thesis, University of Melbourne, 2012

Websites

http://adb.anu.edu.au
www.ancestry.com.au
http://anzacsightsound.org/audios/treating-gallipoli-s-wounded-dr-agnes-bennett
www.awm.gov.au
http://beyond1914.sydney.edu.au

www.buildingsatrisk.org.uk/details/960257
http://cumberbatch.one-name.net
http://ezitis.myzen.co.uk/briefhistoryauxhosps.html
http://Gm1914.wordpress.com/2016/11/10/alice-thomasson/
www.iwm.org.uk
www.gresham.ac.uk/lectures-and-events/the-first-world-war-
    disease-the-only-victor
http://KUMC.edu/wwi/essays-on-first-world-war-medicine/
    index-of-essays/biography/frances-ivens
www.lister-institute.org.uk/about-us/our-heritage
http://maltaramc.com/articles/contents/greatwar.html
www.nwtrcc.org/history/images/1861-hungary.gif
http://nzetc.victoria.ac.nz
www.outskirts.arts.uwa.edu/volumes/volume-7/secomb
www.qaranc.co.uk/voluntary-aid-detachment.php
www.racp.edu.au/www.microbiologysociety.org
www.redcross.org.uk
www.royalherbert.co.uk/history.php
www.ryde.nsw.gov.au
www.samhs.org.au
www.scarletfinders.co.uk
http://sydney.edu.au/medicine/museum/mwmuseum/index.php/
    Early_women_graduates
www.smythe.id.au/diary/ch3.htm
www.thegazette.co.uk
http://trove.nla.gov.au/newspaper
www.vlib.us/medical/gaswar/gas.htm
www.vlib.us/wwi/resources/northseadiary.html#no9

Acknowledgements

Official and public records for the wartime service of the women in this book are almost non-existent and we have relied heavily on rare manuscripts, private papers and memories. Newspaper resources provided by the National Library of Australia's Trove website have been invaluable for this book and all research of women's history in Australia. Sometimes, to our great delight, information has arrived serendipitously.

We wish to acknowledge the hundreds of women doctors throughout the British Empire who replaced their male colleagues when the men departed their positions to enlist with the RAMC or the AAMC. Often they filled medical roles that were previously unattainable to women doctors before the war and demonstrated their professional competence once given the opportunity.

We would like to acknowledge our debt to Dr Ann Mitchell's earlier work on Australia's World War I women doctors; the writings of Dr Leah Leneman and Dr Eileen Crofton on the Scottish Women's Hospitals, Dr Jennian Geddes on the Endell Street Military Hospital; and Dr Jacqueline Healy's work on commemorating women doctors in exhibitions and catalogues at the University of Melbourne Medical History Museum.

We are also grateful for the amazing work on their websites over many years of Jennifer Baker for *Looking for the Evidence*,

Sue Light for *Scarlet Finders* and the creators of *Beyond 1914: The University of Sydney & the Great War*.

We would like to thank Dr Jennian Geddes for informed and eagle-eyed reading and enthusiastic research in England, Dr Ross McMullin for encouragement and valuable editorial advice, and John and Freda Forbes for willing and helpful commentary.

We are very appreciative of the help and encouraging response from the following: William Girling for Dr Katie Ardill (Brice), Graeme Lunn and Dr RCF Stephens for Dr Ethel Baker, Richard Shaw for Dr Rachel Champion (Shaw), Kathy Hancock and Christine McClennan for Dr Mary De Garis, Rob Wagner for Dr Laura Forster, Pacita Alexander for Dr Marjory Little, Christopher McQuellin for Dr Isabel Ormiston, Catherine James Bassett for Dr Vera Scantlebury (Brown), Helen Tuck for Dr Isabella Younger (Ross), and Julianne Richards, Heather Cumming and Marjorie Walker for Sister Elsie Tranter.

We acknowledge the generous permissions of the following:

The text from Vera Brittain's *Chronicle of Youth: The War Diary, 1913–1917* is reproduced by permission of the copyright holders Mark Bostridge and T.J. Brittain-Catlin, Literary Executors for the Estate of Vera Brittain 1970.

The text from the papers of Dr Agnes Bennett is reproduced with the permission of the Alexander Turnbull Library, National Library of New Zealand.

The text from the papers of Dr Eleanor Bourne is reproduced with the permission of the State Library of Queensland.

The text from Eileen Crofton's *The Women of Royaumont* is reproduced with the permission of the Birlinn Publishing Company for Tuckwell Press.

Finally, many thanks for the enthusiasm of our literary agent Margaret Gee and everyone at Penguin Random House.

Index

Discover a
new favourite

Visit **penguin.com.au/readmore**